Gifts of Life

Gifts of Life

Edited by

Deb Stewart

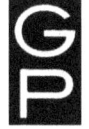

In memory of my sister Laura

24.12.1963–25.12.2006

Gifts of Life
ISBN 978 1 76041 573 0
Copyright © text individual contributors 2007
Copyright © this collection Deb Stewart 2007
Cover image: Deb Stewart

First published 2007
Second edition published 2018

GINNINDERRA PRESS
PO Box 3461 Port Adelaide 5015
www.ginninderrapress.com.au

Contents

Introduction	7
Preface	9
Alison's Story	13
A Carer's Story	16
Care for the Carer	18
A Renal Transplant Patient's Story	21
Ken's Story	24
Sarah's Story of Thanks	28
No Strings Attached	32
Cornea Transplant Story by Kerry Malone	46
Steve's Story	50
Andrew and Alison	52
Laura's Story	56
Margaret Pratt's Story	59
Living Kidney Donor Story – Sue & Vic	61
The Gift of Life – An Organ Donor Saved My Life	63
WOW! – Lisa Upton's Story	66
My Story – Bob Pocock	68
Dylan's Story 18.3.1993–23.10.2005	71
Leonie Ingleton	89
Ebony Keys (poem to an organ donor) – Mel Rees	91

Introduction

Courage and inspiration are what you feel when you read these exceptional stories of everyday families coping with what life has dealt them!

The harsh reality of organ and tissue donation is that we are dealing with life and death!

The courage of donor families at a time of tragedy is magnificent and the inspiration donor families receive at a later time from transplant recipients must truly be the circle of life.

Transplant recipients triumph over numerous and ongoing obstacles but they seem to embrace life in a way that many of us never know! How must it feel to know that someone must die for you to receive an organ transplant?

When our family was faced with our beloved David – brain dead and on life support – the shock and tragedy of what had happened was beyond expression. When asked about donating, his often spoken words came immediately to mind: 'What do you need your organs for when you're dead?'

I encourage you to register.

Visit the website www.davidhookesfoundation.com and follow the online prompts to access the Australian Organ Donor Register; call 1800 777 203; or visit a Medicare office.

Robyn Hookes – 'Organ Donors Give Life!'

Preface

I would like to thank all of the contributors for sharing their courageous and painful, yet hopeful, stories. Thank you also to Robyn Hookes for kindly agreeing to read the manuscript of *Gifts of Life* and write an introduction.

My sister Laura inspired me to bring together these stories in a published collection, so that others may share these experiences and gain an understanding of organ donation from the perspective of both the donor family and the recipient.

Deb Stewart

When you must say 'goodbye' to me
Please do not waste my greatest gift.
Though it is difficult to think of,
My heart can restore life to another
While under earth or flame it will only perish.

My lungs can give someone a chance to simply breathe
Without the aid of oxygen, to move freely
Without the restriction of tubes and cylinders.

Give my kidneys to the dialysis-dependent
So they may be free from hours hooked up to a machine.

My corneas are the gift of sight,
Of colour, light, human faces,
And wonders of nature
To those who have lived in darkness.

My blood should not go to waste
Use it to circulate life in the veins of those in need.

Give my organs as a parting gift to this world
And take comfort in the knowledge that my life has immeasurable worth
Though I may not be particularly gifted or special,
I can share my greatest gift
And feel content, and at peace, to know
That, together, we have given life.

Deb Stewart

Alison's Story

My 18-year-old daughter Alison died in October 1998 from a spontaneous brain haemorrhage caused by a congenital blood vessel malformation that we had no idea she had. I had always considered organ donation as a natural progression if circumstances allowed it, but always in relation to myself – I had never imagined that I would be in a position to make that decision for one of my children. When it happened, it was an easy decision because I had briefly discussed organ donation with Alison when she was going for her learner's permit for her driver's licence. Some good had to come from our dreadful loss and it gives me comfort knowing that her death resulted in six families getting a second chance with their loved one. Nothing could have saved my beautiful girl and I am so proud that we were able to honour her wishes to be an organ donor.

My attitude to a lot of things has changed since losing Alison – I now live my life knowing that life is precious and you don't know what is around the corner. We went to bed one night as a normal family and woke up the next day to our worst nightmare and our lives have been changed immeasurably. We lost one daughter and a few months later discovered that another daughter had the same congenital blood vessel malformation in her brain and she had to have treatment to prevent a similar catastrophe. We also now know that all the next generation will need to be checked when they start to arrive. Our family has been shattered – my marriage broke down and my surviving children have struggled to get through their teens. We are now all sorting ourselves out but it has been a long hard road and there are times when it all comes crashing down again.

In my previous experience working as a nurse, I had been aware of social workers, psychologists and support groups but had always considered them unnecessary – why couldn't people just sort themselves out? When I was confronted with the loss of my daughter, I soon realised that I was going to need help to survive this nightmare and learn to live again. My friends and family were wonderful but there came a time when I felt I was burdening them with too much – I didn't want them feeling guilty that their children were OK and no matter what they said to me they couldn't make it all right again. I spoke to a counsellor and then joined a donor family support group – it was wonderful to be able to listen to other families with similar losses and know that they had survived…somehow. I came to understand that I wasn't going crazy – I was grieving.

I eventually realised that I would never be the same – life would never be the same – but somehow we would get to a stage where we were living a new normal. Part of the journey is coming to terms with the fact that it is OK to feel happiness again. There is so much guilt wrapped up in simple emotions after losing Alison – how dare I laugh when she isn't here to share it? I have accepted that I am forever changed but I also know that it would be a dreadful legacy to her memory for me to waste the rest of my life because of her death. Living my life to the full has to be my tribute to her and my other three children – they should not lose a mother as well as a sister.

Organ donation has been such a positive for me. Alison was a beautiful, loving and wonderful young woman on the brink of her life. She had a lovely boyfriend and they had great plans for the rest of their lives – when they would marry, have their children and all the other myriad plans that young ones make together. Losing Alison has meant the loss of her future – the grandchildren I will never know, the companionship of a daughter to the end of my days. A parent should never have to bury a child.

Knowing that her death resulted in new life for six other people and their families does give me some comfort – it doesn't make it OK that we do not have her with us but I know she would approve that we made the decision to donate her organs. Her liver went to a toddler girl, her lungs went to a teenage girl and her kidneys went to two adults, a male and a female both with families. Her heart could not be transplanted as it was too damaged but her heart valves went to two young women.

I have received letters from some of her recipients and they were just so wonderful to receive. The first letter arrived just after her 19th birthday, some seven months after her death, and it was very emotional but so helpful to know that the toddler girl was doing well. I have since become involved with Transplant Australia and have met many recipients and heard many wonderful stories. It is truly amazing, the miracle of organ donation.

A Carer's Story

Laura (then 38) was diagnosed with primary pulmonary hypertension (PPH) on 27 February 2002. After many hospital visits and tests we were sent to the Alfred Hospital in September for further assessment. We had to fly back to Melbourne the following month and, as Laura was now dependent on oxygen 24 hours a day, special arrangements were put in force with the airline for the transportation of wheelchair and oxygen.

We had accommodation supplied in an apartment about ten minutes walk from the Alfred, with great facilities, complete with kitchen, which allowed me to cook our own meals. Laura was now on the waiting list for a donor organ; she needed a double lung transplant to prolong her life so we were close to the hospital for when the call came. Whilst you are waiting you get into a routine of going out for walks (pushing a wheelchair with oxygen canister attached) shopping and visiting the Alfred for continuing testing and monitoring.

We were fortunate to have friends who lived near Melbourne. They kindly looked after Laura at various times so that I could spend time with my wife back in Adelaide; these were precious times and helped me so much to do what I had to do. During this waiting time we met so many inspirational people, some already transplanted and some waiting. I include as inspiration the many souls who make up the transplant team. You would not want to (or could be) in better hands, no praise is too high and that includes the Adelaide team. I should add that my wife also visited us in Melbourne and that also helped Laura and me.

You get to a point when you just get used to waiting. You do need to bring your sense of humour, be prepared to be calm, have patience, be adaptable – and all that goes for the person being cared for as well! We waited six months and by then her condition had deteriorated so much that she was confined to the hospital and on a very high rate of oxygen. I will never forget the day I was told they had the lungs for her and we went up to the ward to give her the news. The feelings we experienced were many – joy, relief, apprehension, and sadness that a family had lost a loved one but gifted her another chance of life! The surgeons rang me to let me know when each lung had been transplanted and that the procedure had gone well. My wife was by my side when Laura arrived in intensive care; that was late at night and we could only watch as she was on life support, but the next morning, Praise God, she was conscious and able to communicate through pointing out letters on a board. We had been truly blessed and for the next 13 weeks she had regular physio sessions, constant monitoring of her condition and we both had to attend classes dealing with a multitude of aspects concerning transplantation. These classes were a great opportunity to meet and talk with the other recipients and their carers.

My wife and I have been given great peace of mind concerning the events of the past 18 months or so, we believe our faith in Jesus Christ Our Lord has sustained us through this difficult time. Also, prayers from many people all over the world for our daughter, and all the people who have helped her, have been answered!

Care for the Carer

Support books distributed through the hospital support units emphasise the need for carers to take care of themselves and take breaks whenever they can. Reading it, one thinks 'Oh yes' but then that advice seems to get forgotten.

My husband Peter became carer for our daughter Laura, who was diagnosed with PPH and needed a double lung transplant. Her condition had deteriorated so much that it was decided to transfer her to Melbourne to be close to the Alfred Hospital, to be monitored by the transplant team and to await transplant. I was not physically able to care for Laura as she was, by then, in a wheelchair and too heavy for me to push around – so it was logical for Peter to go with her, and I stayed home to arrange the move into the new home we had just completed building – and set up all the jobs associated with that.

Peter and Laura made the move to Melbourne in October 2002. Peter returned home for a few days at the beginning of November, to help me move into our new home. Long-time friends in Melbourne looked after Laura. He also came home for three days to oversee the auction of our old home on 14 December, travelling overnight on the Overland and arriving home about an hour before the auction time of 12 o'clock. He was totally exhausted!

When he went back to Melbourne we kept in touch most days by telephone – we took the precaution of arranging for Telstra to cap our call costs to $1.50 to enable us to have long conversations – to help and encourage one another.

The next time I saw him was on 31 December 2002, when he came home for a surprise visit. He was given a lift from the airport by a friend, who had kept the secret. The doorbell rang – I was having dinner and feeling very lonely! What a wonderful surprise! However, I was horrified to see how thin and ill he looked. He just collapsed into my arms, he was unable to walk unassisted. He has always been physically strong but the emotion of being apart from me was as draining as all the work he now had to do as Laura's carer. He stayed home for four days and recouped some of his strength.

In Melbourne his days consisted of preparing all the meals, doing the washing, and shopping. He also had to ensure that Laura was up and ready for the constant round of hospital appointments, and push her there in the wheelchair. It was also down to him to encourage Laura, who was separated from her two young sons and missing them. He would push her around Albert Park every day.

Obviously, due to her condition, Laura suffered emotionally as well and there would sometimes be inevitable tension between them. Both say that it was only their sense of humour that got them through each day.

In February Laura was admitted to hospital to have a pump fitted and to be trained to administer Prostacyclin. Peter took the opportunity to come home, having arranged for friends at his church to visit Laura each day – thank God for those wonderful people.

Even at home, Peter kept in constant touch with the hospital staff regarding the treatment. He was home for three weeks and then returned to be trained in the administration of the drug. However, Laura's condition was deteriorating at a rapid rate of knots and she was not released from the hospital. During this time Peter was visiting her several times a day, as well as keeping up with the washing etc.

March 31 dawned; Peter was up early as he was going to see the transplant staff concerning an incident which had occurred over the weekend. This incident had caused Laura a great deal of trauma, which in turn affected Peter. However, when he arrived at the hospital he was met by the transplant coordinator, who advised him that a donor had been found and Laura would be having surgery soon. Everything else was forgotten!

I travelled over that same afternoon on the first flight I could get; I arrived at their apartment at 8.30 p.m. just before he received a phone call to say that the first lung had been transplanted and they were about to start the second. I was glad to be there, to be together and support each other at this time. We were elated when the second phone call came to say the surgery was complete – doctors were amazed at how easily and quickly everything went. A miracle! We were able to visit Laura at about midnight in ICU.

I was able to stay with Peter for three weeks to look after him and to visit Laura each day. Her recovery during that time was not without problems, but we were able to help and support each other. During this time our youngest daughter also came over and gave us both a boost.

Laura was still in hospital when I returned home – three months intensive physio was ahead of her before she could return to Adelaide.

I was able to visit again for a week at the beginning of June. This time when Peter met me near the hospital I was devastated to see how thin he was – almost skeletal. I realised that, although I had been visiting, he had not had a proper break away from his Melbourne routine for about four months. He was physically and emotionally spent.

Peter and Laura returned to Adelaide on 30 June 2003 – needless to say, we were all delighted to have them home. Laura was able to cope at home with just occasional help from us with the jobs she was not able to manage.

Coming home was traumatic for Peter in as much as 'home' was not the home he left when he went to Melbourne. Although he had visited me, it had been like a holiday he said; now it was home but it didn't feel like it. Everything was strange – he felt he didn't belong. After about three weeks TLC he started to resemble his old self. He'd put on weight and enjoyed being home. However, he couldn't face the volunteer work that he had done for years prior to leaving for Melbourne and he felt useless.

I'm sure this would be considered normal, as for 24 hours a day, seven days a week he had been tuned in to Laura's needs and suddenly it had ended.

Carers: YOU are every bit as important as the patient. Take breaks as often as you can – if you don't have family to help out, find a good local church or carers' support group. Let them know your situation; they will lift and encourage you and ease the burden. When you are refreshed you are able to better cope with the demands on you. God bless you. Valerie.

A Renal Transplant Patient's Story

♥

My name is Twanny Farrugia and I was born in the Mitarfa Military Hospital in Malta in the early 1950s. For the first 11 years of my life, I lived in Rahal Ghdid. These were the happiest years of my life. Unbeknown to me and my family, I had a time bomb ticking away inside of me, ready to blow up and not only possibly kill me but alter my whole family's life.

It was 1969 when I was diagnosed with renal failure after a lifetime of undiagnosed illness. I was fortunate that my parents decided to immigrate to Australia as this proved a life-saving exercise for me. Malta at that stage did not have a renal unit as advanced as here in Australia. Renal failure was the unknown time bomb ticking away inside of me for most of my life. If this had gone untreated, it would have had terrible consequences for my family. I would have died. As it was, even with this diagnosis, life for the next few years was going to be a battle for my family, my friends, health service providers and of course myself. Furthermore, it was to leave many physical and psychological scars not only for myself but also for all those loving and supporting me. However, as you can see, I survived.

At age 15, I collapsed and was transported to the casualty department of St Vincent's Hospital in Melbourne. This was the start of a nightmare which was to conclude happily in being transplanted on 22–23 October 1971. Apart from dialysis and transplantation, this passage of chronic illness was to encompass a multitude of other ailments ranging from mobility, heart attacks to vision impairment and many other health issues.

Eighteen months after being admitted to hospital, four arteriovenous fistulas were performed, one of which was successful and was utilised throughout my dialysing period, while the others were inoperative from the start. A fistula is a medical procedure where the surgeon (under general anaesthetic) joins a vein (slow-flowing blood) to an artery (fast-flowing blood). Then, a few days after the operation, the veins on your arm will grow bigger and the more you use the arm later on the better. The size of the cut to make a fistula is about eight centimetres long and there will be a small scar afterwards. This procedure allows an access site for dialysing.

In the late 60s and early 70s, dialysis consisted of six to eight hours three times a week depending on height, weight and overall health. The machine used was a Drake Willock and given that I was a very small specimen (weight approximately three to four stone and four feet 10 inches tall), I used to be completely drained after a dialysis session.

Overall, even though dialysis was a painful process for me as an individual, it was also a reasonably happy period of my life. The main reason being that dialysis was still a reasonably new therapy strategy and renal units were not as overcrowded as they appear to be today. Having one-on-one nursing care also proved less stressful than it is today, where one nurse and or technician may be caring for up to eight patients at a time.

Notwithstanding the excellent medical care, I would not be alive today if it was not for the donor family and for the magnificent unconditional love and support I received from my family, friends and all the staff involved at the hospital in Melbourne. Overriding all this, the main reason for surviving life in general and my health problems in particular was and still is my faith in God, as I perceive him, followed by my own family, donor family, friends and the medical profession (not necessarily in that order).

Having been given this precious gift of life I have endeavoured to contribute back to the community which has given me so much in life. I have participated in the Dialysis and Transplant Association (a self-help group) basically from its early beginnings. My affiliation with DATA spans approximately 30 years (as president, vice president, secretary, and as an executive and general committee member) while concurrently spending 25 years with Kidney Health Australia, for which both organisations have presented me with honorary life memberships. Furthermore, during this same 30-year period, I have been and still am a volunteer with various welfare organisations.

Socially, my health issues have not stopped me from leading a reasonably active life. I enjoy ballroom dancing (ex-competitor and medallist), lawn bowls (ex-competitor), cycling, reading, music, meeting people and socialising with my friends, while endeavouring to enjoy life in general.

In conclusion, I wish to take this opportunity to again thank my family who have supported me throughout life, warts and all. Also, thanks must go to the donor family who during the loss of their loved one considered offering that most precious gift – the gift of life – together with my friends and the medical fraternity. In 1984 and 1995, on the death of my father and brother respectively, I became aware of the meaning of becoming a donor family. My family feels that the scales have now been balanced. I received the the gift of life and our family members returned that gift of life to others. The circle has now been completed.

I hope this story will encourage people to become both organ and blood donors as, without these types of donors, I would have been dead long ago. To donate organs you can contact Kidney Health Australia via their website www.kidney.org.au or phone (03) 9674 4300. For blood donation, contact the Australian Red Cross Blood Bank on http://www.donateblood.com.au or 131 495.

Ken's Story

In 1994 my family and I moved to Melbourne from Adelaide. This move occurred as a result of a restructure in the organisation I was working for at the time. When I started work in Melbourne, I discovered there was a gym at my workplace and decided to join up. Part of the membership process was to have a medical examination, which required a blood pressure check. I was advised that my blood pressure was a little high – 150/90 – probably the result of starting a new job. After a few weeks, however, it did not come down and I was sent to a GP for examination. He put me on blood pressure tablets and began a series of tests. The end result of these tests was that I was diagnosed with IgG nepthropathy, an auto-immune disease that was attacking my kidneys and causing my increased blood pressure.

The formal medical advice was that there was no treatment to stop the disease but it may stop by itself, or it may get worse and I could end up on dialysis. This came as a big shock as, until this time, I had been very healthy and had little involvement with the medical system. The good news I was told was that blood pressure tablets would control my blood pressure, which would minimise kidney damage and prolong the life of my kidneys. This was the beginning of a 10-year journey through the medical system and the management of a chronic disease.

Over the next few years I found that my blood pressure was very unstable and the only advice from doctors was to take more and more blood pressure tablets. I was not happy with the advice I was receiving and the side effects from blood pressure tablets so I decided to consult some alternative therapy practitioners. They were not able to cure my condition but were very helpful in educating me about managing my health.

By 1999 my disease had progressed and it became evident that I would end up on dialysis. During the years preceding 1999 I had regular blood tests, which indicated my kidney function was deteriorating. As it is a slow process, you don't really notice the physical impact it has on your day to day life. I really became aware of it when my family and I went for a mild bush walk and I found I had no energy and had to return to the car.

In 1999, my wife and I attended a dialysis education session at the hospital. We were told about haemodialysis and peritoneal dialysis, both of which were frightening prospects. At the time it was difficult to take in the implications of what it means to your lifestyle.

In April 2001 I started dialysis at the Royal Melbourne Hospital. This was a very difficult experience. I felt shocking after the experience and there was nothing except one shared TV to watch during the treatment. The following day I felt as though I had been drinking heavily the night before. I was fortunate that my employer allowed me time off during the week with no impact on my salary.

In 2003 my younger brother, Michael, rang me from Adelaide, while I was on dialysis, to offer me a kidney. This was earth-shattering news and I looked forward to a transplant possibly six months later, after completion of all the tests. Unfortunately the six months turned into two years, but in early 2005 I received an email from my brother indicating that all tests were passed and that he was happy to proceed. I felt like I had won the lottery, finally an escape from the grind of dialysis three times per week, at four hours per session.

In March 2005 I flew to Adelaide, where my brother and I met with the transplant coordinator at the Queen Elizabeth Hospital, a wonderful woman. She showed us a video that described the transplant process and gave interviews with a few people who had gone through the process. At this meeting my brother and I agreed that the operation should be in Adelaide as he lived there and he wanted keyhole surgery, which was not common in Melbourne. This form of surgery would greatly reduce the recovery time for him. Then she asked us to nominate a date for the operation. After due consideration, we all agreed on Wednesday 13 July. I flew back to Melbourne and told my family that the date had been set for the operation. My wife and I agreed that the whole family should be in Adelaide for the operation and we commenced the planning.

We arrived in Adelaide approximately 10 days prior to the operation, as we had to settle in to our rented accommodation and go through some final review processes at the hospital. The final meeting prior to the operation was for myself and family, and my brother and his family, to meet the surgeon and senior doctor to review the operations and risk. Although I had been waiting for this for two years, it suddenly became very real and stressful. The thought of taking a working part from another person's body was difficult to come to terms with. I could easily understand if he had changed has mind about donating at the last minute.

At 4 p.m. on 12 July, we checked into the hospital. I had a pick line put in my neck and both families went out for dinner. The dinner began for me with two Scotch and dries; it was a very tense affair as we all contemplated the risks of the days and weeks ahead. I slept poorly that night thinking of what lay ahead and hearing the noises of people walking in the corridors.

On Wednesday I went to visit my brother early in the morning to see how he felt, was he still comfortable to go ahead. (I could easily understand someone changing his or her mind at the last minute.) At about 10 a.m. my family came to see me and we chatted until the nurse came in and said, 'Mr Pedlow, it's time to go.' After what seemed a long wait, the surgeon came to see us and advised that my brother's kidney had been successfully removed. He was doing fine and they were ready to commence my operation.

From that point on I do not remember a thing until I woke up in my room surrounded by my family and the nurse. On waking I remember thinking that nothing was hurting too much and being relieved that the operation had been successful. For approximately 48 hours following the operation I had a dedicated nurse in my room in case of complications.

Thankfully there were no complications and I slowly recovered over the next five days. Whilst I was happy that my operation was successful, I was also concerned how my brother was recovering. It was very important to me that both he and I regained full health and that there were no side effects from the operation. In my brother's case, keyhole surgery had been used to remove the kidney, which theoretically meant a shorter recovery. Due to the nature of the operation he was in significant pain after the operation but this was managed and he was able to leave hospital on the Friday, two days after the operation. This is a great improvement on other removal methods where the incision is large and the hospital stay is at least seven days.

I left hospital six days after my operation and, whilst the care of the staff had been great, I was happy to be leaving. To walk outside (albeit slowly) and feel the wind on my face was tremendous. I felt as though I had successfully climbed the mountain and was now heading home. In the middle of September I was feeling fairly healthy so I decided to go for a day of snow skiing. I started very cautiously and during the day steadily increased the effort. I found that I got far less tired skiing after the transplant than previously when I was on dialysis.

As I recovered from the operation I began to contemplate what the future held, no more dialysis, no diet restrictions, and another 15 hours in a week to do with as I pleased. The future looked very good. Whilst dialysis is a life-saving process it does have a massive impact on your life in terms of the time it takes and your physical well being after the treatment. In my case it meant getting home at 9 p.m. on Tuesdays and Thursdays, I would work from 8.30 to 3 then go and have dialysis from 4 to 8. On Saturday I would get up at 5.15 a.m. so that I could start dialysis at 6.30 a.m. finishing at 10.30 a.m. I would get home at about midday and often have a nap in the afternoon, as the dialysis left me very tired. The net result was, in effect, that you had one day on the weekend to do what you wanted rather than two. Another benefit would be going on holidays without first having to check if dialysis was available and, if so, if I could book in. All of this took a lot of time away from me and imposed more work on my wife.

In closing I would like to thank my brother for making this most generous gift and to the transplant team at the Queen Elizabeth Hospital in Adelaide who do such a marvellous job.

Sarah's Story of Thanks

My name is Sarah and this is a story of thanks. I am 29 years old and my father received a double lung transplant in 2003. He was sick from when I was 10 or 11 years old. At first the doctors thought he was suffering from asthma. I remember that he couldn't breathe as easily as he used to and he wasn't really playing with me any more. After being diagnosed with asthma, they thought that Dad had emphysema, but much later he was diagnosed with a genetic lung deficiency, although this was kept from me for quite a while.

My earlier memories are of Dad having shortness of breath, not being able to walk as far as he used to, and an increasing number of puffer's and medications to make it a little easier for him. I found my diary from when I was a teenager and found these entries:

> Saturday 20 August 1994: This was a really bad day today, it was scaring me and I think it really has hit me now, how sick he is getting. I think it's the first time I cried like I did today. It was scary, it really was. I hope to God he will let him be and make him well again.
>
> Sunday 30 October 1994: Dad found it hard getting on the plane to Cairns today, Megan cried.

The next few years were long and slow as Dad deteriorated. At first the use of puffers helped, then the use of a nebuliser helped. At first Dad could still do things around the house but in the end just walking a few steps was too much effort, getting out of the car or bed could take 15 to 20 minutes. My heart broke when Dad couldn't utter an answer to a question, because he was too exhausted, and his temper flared because he was so frustrated. I remember changing washers in taps and cementing and all those traditional

Dad jobs. I remember crying to myself because I just wanted to leave and see my friends but I had to get wood inside or do gardening, or fix something. My heart would almost burst out of my chest in frustration, but I always bit my tongue and got on with it. Looking back now, it gave me strength of character, but then it was hard and felt cruel.

Holidays were heartbreaking because Dad couldn't go out, or only for a short while. Dad used to dance with Mum for half a dance at weddings (it was all he could muster), but in the end Mum had to go to them alone with us kids. I used to watch her eyes well with tears watching other couples dance. Mum, by this time, was socialising completely alone, when we felt safe leaving Dad.

Memories of my childhood with Dad well are very few. In fact, I can't remember any, I can only remember the stress and tears and tablets and puffers. The sound of a puffer sends a chill down my spine to this day.

Jealousy played a big part in my life. I was jealous of my friends for having healthy families and I was mad at the world for tearing my family apart like this. I would cry silently at night and wake up with the strong face that helped me through the day and helped Mum through hers.

Becoming an adult, the truth came to me, a realisation that my father was slowly dying. Many nights I would cry after saying goodnight to him.

We knew a transplant was the only way that he was going to live, but Dad had not put himself on the active list and we were wondering when he would. One day my sister told Dad she was waiting until he was better before she was going to have a baby. That was enough to get him straight on that active list. He was on the list for about three weeks when I was sitting with my boyfriend at his house and he handed me a newspaper article. It was the beginning of Organ Donation Week and there was a story on average waiting periods for organs. I read the average waiting period for lungs was nine to 12 months. I cried, I knew we didn't have that long. I said goodbye and drove home upset. I got home and said hi to Mum and walked into Dad's room. He was awake and it was almost 8.45 p.m., very late for him. I said my hellos and had a shower. After that I chatted with Dad for a little bit.

Dad's mobile phone rang at 9.18 p.m. exactly; we looked at each other and knew what it was. Dad asked me to get it – I said no. Dad answered it, I heard 'hospital' and 'Sydney' and I knew what it was. I ran to get Mum and said, 'I think it's Dad's lungs, Mum.' We all panicked, as Dad hung up the phone he said, 'I love you' to the nurse and cried. In an enormous rush we managed to get Dad and a half-packed case into the car. I drove them to the Royal Flying Doctors and a nurse and pilot were waiting for us. It took about 15 minutes to get him on the gurney, as he couldn't breathe laying on his back and had to be strapped in the fetal position like a sick little child. I cried as I saw him for what I thought might be the last time. I had thoughts in my head of my sister not being able to ever see him again, as I couldn't contact her, much as I tried. We wheeled him to the plane and I hugged my mum goodbye. My dad looked so sick; he didn't look like he could survive the flight, let alone the surgery. He was so little and was trying to be so brave; I kissed him and told him I couldn't watch him going on the plane. He groaned, 'I'll see you soon' and I kissed him on the head. I walked away and thought it may just have been the last time I had seen my dad. I eventually got hold of Megan when I was driving home. She cried that she was meant to be going (she was Mum's support person).

I cried most of the night. My Auntie and uncle stayed with me and I lit the candle Dad had asked me to and it stayed lit for his entire surgery. I cried for all the years we had lost, and all the years we may lose, I cried because it might be the end. I cried because maybe all those years weren't that bad, because I could still see him and talk to him and tell him I loved him. I wanted to just tell him one more time. We were waiting and waiting and as time went on I realised the reality of all of this, someone had just lost someone that they loved. The start of our miracle was the beginning of their nightmare.

I didn't cry as much as I thought I would when I first saw Dad walking towards me, although I did hug him too tight. He was standing straight and wasn't hunched over gasping for air; it was what I always thought my dad should be. I couldn't remember him like this but I knew he was like this before his sickness. I watched everything in amazement, the way he breathed and walked, the way his voice was so strong, and the way he held Mum's hand as they walked, yes walked, to the hospital. I felt selfish because I felt that Dad had got what he deserved, another chance at life.

It has been a long and winding road. Dad works a few hours a week now and enjoys the challenge, he has setbacks, and we still have times his health scares us, but ups and downs are life's little lessons. I fret if Dad coughs or needs to walk up stairs and he tells me he's fine.

My parents get to know each other more; they go shopping, to the movies, even a coffee together is special to them. It's special to all my family, brothers and sisters, nieces and nephews.

I never thought my dad would walk me down the aisle, or hold my babies, or be able to teach me through my life. I realise now as a grown adult with a partner and a house, and bills to pay, how I learnt at such a young age the lesson that people usually learn when they are much older, that sometimes there are things you will never have control of, and all you can do is ride the wave until it ends, good or bad.

We all learnt that the people you tend to neglect are those you should cherish the most, and that you can be the most thankful you can ever be to someone you can never meet, and a family you can never thank in person. This has been a miracle and will never be forgotten.

I am thankful for my experiences and I look back and I am proud of myself. I am proud of my sister. I am proud of my dad. But especially, I am proud of my mum. Not every woman would stick around for almost 20 years going through what she went through. It would've been easier to leave but she loved that man more than she ever knew. We will never forget how lucky we are.

No Strings Attached

On 17 November 1999, my brother Hayden received a new kidney; his own were failing due to nephritis. I was the donor, and if this story helps someone else through the process of becoming a donor, or encourages someone else to do the same thing, then I will feel as though I have done a little bit to help. I have a young family and run a family business with my husband Grant, so I am no different from most of the people out there. I have no special gifts or qualities that made me able to do this, the only quality that I consider relevant is that I was willing.

September 1998

I was down in the shearing shed when I heard the mobile ringing in the car. Hayden had been in Adelaide to see a specialist. The outcome of this appointment was that he would need a transplant in the next 18 months to two years. Of course he was devastated and upset. My first reaction and comment was 'Don't worry, you can have one of mine.' I never thought twice about it. Emma, Hayden's partner, contacted the doctor to inform him of my choice and idea and that started the ball rolling. It seemed to roll very slowly, but roll it did.

January 1999

I received a letter from Hayden's doctor today informing me to go to my local GP for a blood test so that a cross match can be done. I went to see Dr Davies almost straight away. He advised me to go to RPH (Royal Perth Hospital) as, being in the country, it would make the blood another 12 to 18 hours old before testing. He was very supportive of my decision. Dr Davies rang RPH and found out what I had to do and where to go.

February 1999

I am off to RPH for my blood to be taken. Hayden and Emma are in Adelaide for the same test. Dr Thomas came out and spoke to me, he asked many questions and went on to tell me that I couldn't just walk in and become a donor. I was asked to join the program at RPH and attend clinic on a Tuesday. My first impression of Dr Thomas isn't good.

March 1999

Dr Thomas asked more questions did all the routine things, blood pressure etc. I was then sent down to the blood room to be tested for everything and I mean everything! I also had to fill out a form on my history. I now have to say that my first impression of Dr Thomas was wrong and I'm glad that he will be my doctor. I feel very comfortable with him and like his directness.

Emma rang today with the test results. I was almost too scared to ask, I so much wanted to do this. YES YES YES! It did turn out to be in my favour. Thank God.

There have been so many offers of support through this whole process; it's been just amazing. There have also been some unexpected reactions. Some really surprised me. Jackson is one of my sons; he is seven years old and has shown a real interest in all the gory bits. He wants to know where I'll be cut and how many stitches. Breanna is three years old and really isn't that interested at all. She just thinks it's wonderful going to stay with Grant's parents while I travel to RPH and also she is quite young. Craig is one of my stepsons, he is 21 years old and thinks it's great that I'm trying to be a donor for Hayden. Ben is 18, he is my other stepson. Ben's reaction surprised me – he said he was worried and didn't know if he could do it if needed. I talked to him about this and said that it was a very personal thing and it was something I felt very positive about. I believe it is up to the individual it doesn't mean you're bad if you can't for whatever reason it may be. At end of the day you have to be comfortable with the choice you make.

Mum and Dad must be worried sick. I can't imagine what they're going through. Grant, my husband, has been supportive but is also worried. I have a really good feeling about this and believe with all my heart that it will work out and be successful. When I got my tissue test results back I thought that was it! I was going to be the donor! I was told I had just run the first metre of a 100-metre race and I still had a long way to go yet. It is a race I plan to run and win for both my brother and myself and win I will. Pig-headed is something I am and until a test shows differently I will believe that I'll be the donor. The one thing I have learned is to trust my gut feeling. I'm here for the long haul.

July 1999

I received a letter today from Hayden's doctor informing me that his condition has deteriorated and the time has come to start planning for the transplant. I can't imagine what he is going through. I cried when I read the letter – not for me but for Hayden and how sick he is.

I've attended clinic today. I was running late and got held up in traffic. I missed Dr Thomas, so I waited quite some time before seeing another doctor. He wanted me to redo tests and as he wasn't sure of what was going on. This made me feel quite uneasy but I did go down to blood room and had all sorts of vials filled with blood for different tests. I also enquired about having my next set of tests done sooner but was told 10.8.99 was quite quick, two weeks away and there was no way I could have them sooner. I spoke to Hayden and Emma tonight and told them that today was a complete waste of time, my fault for being late so nothing was gained at all really.

I spoke to Hayden today he is really concerned about the effects this will have on my life later. I told him it is something I really want to do. I would be fine in the long term, in the short term there would be recovery, but after that I would be doing all that I do now. Somehow I got the feeling he didn't believe me and I do understand that he is worried, but my thoughts are if I'm not why should you be? It will all be fine – I have a great feeling about all this and will do all that I can to help him as I know he would for me. There must be so much going through his mind, not only his own health problems but also thinking of how this will all affect me in the long run.

August 1999

I have just seen Dr Thomas and been to the blood room for more tests. I've also had my kidneys ultrasounded. The nighties they make you put on for these tests are so degrading, it reduced me to tears. I felt horrible. The ultrasound seemed to go well. My kidneys look good, but I won't have test results for some time, about two weeks. I also had a spiral CT scan that was weird – they put some kind of fluid into your veins (via a needle near your wrist) and then took pictures of my kidneys and other organs. The fluid gave a weird sensation like you were wetting yourself – luckily the nurses warned me of this, as I would have really panicked. It was about 4.30 p.m. before I left hospital, long day. I always seem to feel so lonely in the hospital. Never mind, today's over and I just have to wait for the test results. I feel I've spent so much time waiting – it's all you seem to do. I really feel for my brother, he now has a yucky rash on top of everything else. Apparently it comes with renal failure. He is also vomiting a lot and not sleeping well due to getting up all through the night for the toilet, he's getting sick quick, losing weight and so on.

Hayden and Emma have been back to the specialist in Adelaide. They've received a written statement on the results of tests and have set an operation date 15.9.99, but won't confirm it till they receive the film from my tests so they can view the organ. Apparently all looks fine except that it looks like I have a two-centimetre adenoma on my left adrenal gland.

Well it's now been decided that they won't operate on the 15.9.99 as they still don't have the film from my test results. I feel really annoyed and frustrated. Hayden is really suffering yet he still manages to work somehow. They are talking about operating on 20.10.99. This would suit me, as I'd like to be around for my daughter's fourth birthday.

September 1999

Well, it's been cancelled again. The growth I have on my Adrenal gland has to be investigated further to rule out cancer, although my doctor still believes it is a non-functioning growth not cancer. I am not worried at all and believe it is just a growth and that's all, just a hiccup. I'm in clinic again now waiting to see Dr Thomas.

I've had to collect urine for 48 hours for this test. I was so scared coming here that I would drop it and the container split or something (just my luck!). It's actually quite heavy.

I finally got in to see Dr Thomas and he still believes it will all be fine. My blood pressure is great as usual and he was sad for me that the operation had been cancelled again but wished me all the best and again congratulated me on my decision to be a donor. He has being great through all of this, very helpful and very easy to get in contact with.

October 1999

Well we have a confirmed date, 17.11.99. This is later than I ever thought and it will now be much harder for Grant and his parents with the kids. This is the start of harvest. It's flat out but I'm not complaining – we've got a date that's confirmed at last!

My test results are back and it appears to be a non-functioning adenoma just above my left kidney. They have decided to remove this with the kidney during the operation. I am trying to get organised in the office and house. Jackson is really worried now and also quite clingy. Breanna is excited about going to stay out the farm, not at all concerned, so that's good. The boys are very supportive but are concerned also. I'm excited that it is all starting to fall into place. Grant is worried but very supportive and said he'd do the same.

I've had a call from Adelaide from the liaison officer in the renal unit to get accommodation organised and also get a ticket booked for the plane flight. They have informed me that I must be there the week before the operation. I hadn't planned on that and don't want to go that early but have to have more tests done in Adelaide. I thought I had already had them done.

I still believe it's more important that Grant stay with the kids than travel with me, as much as I'd like it. They will really need him at this time especially, Jackson being that bit older and understanding so much more. He came home from the farm the other day most concerned and asked all these gory questions. After it all I asked what had made him ask them again. His reply was he'd just seen them remove the kidneys from a sheep and all of a sudden all he could think of was me having the operation. I then had to really explain in great detail what was going to happen and reassure him that I was going to be treated very differently than a sheep being killed for meat (farm kids!). I was only having one kidney removed and would be fine in no time. Although he had watched this process many times he had never taken much notice of the organs being removed but all of a sudden there was a connection. After we spoke about it in great detail he was fine.

9.11.99

I'm running around like a chook with its head cut off making sure everything is done. The local paper rang late this afternoon to ask if they could come out and do an article on the transplant. I said no as I'm leaving tomorrow and it's just too much. I want to be with my family now, they understood and will ring after I return.

10.11.99

I had a good flight but I was shocked and saddened to hear that Hayden has been admitted to Royal Adelaide and is now in complete renal failure.

11.11.99

I was up early to go into hospital to see Hayden this morning with Emma. We had to wait to see him as he'd been taken into theatre to have a shunt put in. It was about 9.30 a.m. before I saw him. I couldn't stop crying when I saw him, he is so sick. I couldn't stop holding him. I can't believe they let him go this far without doing something about it. I was shocked, I never imagined for one minute he was this bad. He never complained. I thought my being a donor would stop him reaching the bottom but it didn't work that way. I left there and went to QEII Hospital where the transplant is going to take place. On my arrival I was informed there was a 60% chance the transplant will be cancelled as it looks like Hayden needs a blood transfusion. In that case it will be three weeks before they will operate at the earliest. I don't want this cancelled. Hayden is really upset about the news. I've just had my ECG and also a chest X-ray and met the surgeon who will perform the operation. His name is Dr Rao and he seems to be a bit hopeful so fingers crossed.

Still no news as to whether the operation is cancelled or not. I'll have to go home if it is I can't stay that long (three weeks) and then return when they can operate. I really believe deep down it will go ahead.

12.11.99

Hayden has dialysis again today and I have a glucose test to be done at QEII and to see Dr Rao as well. I also have to watch a video on the operation with Toni, the very nice liaison nurse. It's now nearly lunch time and still no word on the operation. I keep telling myself that no news is good news. I've seen the video, the operation looked good, not too bad and the pain thing doesn't bother me. Neither does the wound when and if I ever get it. I wish someone could tell me how Hayden is going and if he's any better this morning. I'm starting to feel very lonely now here.

The doctors rang mid-afternoon to confirm the operation. YEE-HAA! It will go ahead. We were all so relieved to hear the news.

Sadly it didn't last long, we were all laughing and really happy that it was happening when the hospital rang me to say that the glucose test would have to be repeated first thing Monday morning as I'm borderline. What does that mean? Bad by the sound of it. It's Friday afternoon and I now have to wait all weekend before any further decision is made, so again we don't know what's going on. I'm really scared now that it will be cancelled for good and another donor will have to be found. I can't imagine what Hayden and Emma are thinking right now. I really want to do this, it has to be me, I have to keep positive, it will be me, please let it be me. Why does all this uncertainty keep cropping up. It's really making me nervous.

15.11.99

Back into hospital this morning bright and early for a tissue test and to redo the glucose test. Hayden was supposed to dialyse at 8.30 this morning but it was 11.30 a.m. before they had him hooked up. He is having trouble getting around now due to the gout in his foot. This must be frustrating for him – it is for me and I'm only watching.

I'm sitting in pre-admission writing this and still waiting for the glucose results. I've never been so nervous before, it has to be okay. I've spoken to a nurse and anaesthetists; this could take up to three hours they told me. I'm getting used to waiting.

I have received my glucose results, they are now going to cross match them more because they seem to be so low. Well I'm out of pre admission and Hayden has finished dialyses and is at the dentist. They won't operate unless all dental work is done due to infection after operation. I've been here since 7.30 this morning and it's now 5 p.m. Still waiting to hear back about the glucose test.

Well, I have heard now and I am to repeat it tomorrow morning again. All I want to do now is go and ring Grant and the kids. They aren't aware of all this with the operation still not being confirmed.

16.11.99

Having glucose redone, the nurses in the blood room are now calling me a pincushion. It is really starting to hurt now, my arms are bruised and sore big time. I have to sit here in the blood room for several hours and have blood taken every hour to watch the levels after taking the glucose drink. It is so boring, Mum and Dad float in and out and keep me company and I even managed to find a book to read.

Well that's all finished now, only waiting for results again. I really don't know what I will do if it isn't in my favour and the operation is cancelled. I still have to go to St Andrews for more testing and needles (angiogram and MRI) but I'm nearly there. With a bit of luck, tomorrow at this time my operation will be over and this will all be history.

Mum, Dad and Emma have gone home for the night but they will be back in the morning. I've asked that they don't come in before the operation and see me as it would be too teary and I'm to go in at about 7.30 tomorrow morning. I've spent a few hours with Hayden he is also relieved but very nervous about it all. I'm actually excited and feeling really positive. We had lots of laughs about different things and also shed lots of tears. He is so grateful, it is really overwhelming. All I want at the end of this is for him to have his health as without that you have nothing in life really.

19.11.99

I'm sore and very tender but the painkillers are doing a good job. Dad, Mum, Emma, Becky and Marg have been with me off and on since coming out of recovery. I don't really remember too much but I feel good about it all. I haven't seen Hayden yet but have been given lots of messages from him. He is doing really well, he came out of the operation feeling better and looking better already. That's amazing as I feel like I've been hit by a truck! I'm very slow moving and tender, I would have liked to have seen Hayden yesterday but just couldn't get out of bed. Just trying to get to the toilet was a big thing; let alone down to his room. (It would have been nice to have the catheter a bit longer but they removed that yesterday in high dependency along with the drain that was in my side near my hip.)

I'm waiting for someone to come and pick me up in the wheelchair to see Hayden as there's no way I could walk that far on my own. Like I said, getting to the toilet-bathroom is like winning a marathon, though I must admit I'm in a ward with five other ladies. No joke, I must be the youngest by 60 years (I'm 27). They all seem nice and their families are in and out all the time so I'm actually feeling like I'm doing really well as I can get out of bed even if it does take a while and a bit of sweating.

Well I've just returned from being with Hayden and he looks great. I've spent the best part of the day with him, we had lots of laughs and it is just amazing how well he looks. He said he feels good. The doctors said they're trying to slow the kidney down as it is working flat out and producing 24 litres of urine in 24 hours so they are busy keeping the fluid up to him. Up until this point he has been on a restricted amount of fluid per day but now he can't drink enough.

When anyone goes to see Hayden they have to put gloves and a gown on due to the risk of infection. I'm now really uncomfortable and want to sleep, I feel exhausted.

20.11.99

Doctor came in this morning and said I can go back to the unit. I don't feel that I'm ready to go yet but they know best, I hope.

I'm now back at the unit but Hayden isn't doing very well. He's starting to reject. He's upset and worried but I still believe it will be fine, it's just another hiccup. I don't think it helps me being around at the moment as I'm still finding it very hard to move around and it's a reminder to him of what I did and he doesn't need that. He has to concentrate on himself and not worry about me; he has to stay positive, he really needs Emma not me. I won't go in to the hospital tomorrow, they now think that the kidney has been damaged by up to 20% and he is really upset and angry.

We all went to Emma's parents for tea tonight. I don't have much of an appetite, as I feel really bloated all the time. I have these pains under my shoulders, which the doctor said is the gas that they use during the operation lodging in there. I still look as if I'm pregnant, really bloated (swelling and so on from the operation – thank god for track pants and big jumpers) but the swelling in my face has gone down. It does hurt or ache a lot under my shoulders; they've said it will pass in a few days.

21.11.99

I've spent the day at the unit with Dad in the morning while Mum was at the hospital and vice versa in the afternoon. I didn't go to see him. I wanted to but he doesn't need me in there. They still aren't sure about the rejection and I'm still not moving well and at times am uncomfortable. I'm now only taking Panadeine Forte and I'm feeling much stronger today although I got out of bed the wrong way this morning and felt like I was going to faint. I should have just asked for help, ah that would be too easy for me. My shoulders aren't as sore as they were but I'm still really bloated (only looking eight months pregnant now not 10).

22.11.99

I feel stronger and better today, still tender but it's easier to move around. Bit by bit I'll get there. I went and spent time with Hayden today. He is feeling a bit better and it looks like there's no damage to the kidney and they now have the rejection sorted out. Apparently you should expect rejection in some form big or small. It's looking good again. Emma is a real hero in all this, her support to Hayden is fantastic and she stays positive even when she's not really feeling that way herself. Hayden looks to her for that at times and gets great comfort from it. I'm not so bloated today and my shoulders aren't as sore either, looking only about six months pregnant now.

23.11.99

I feel really good today, stronger and not as tender. I'm still taking Panadeine Forte. I went and saw the doctor at Queen Elizabeth. Mr Rao, the surgeon, was happy with everything and removed one stitch that was really annoying me where the drain was, just beside my hip. He said that all the other stitches should dissolve. I even went shopping with Mum and Dad. I think the more I move the better. The doctor also said I can fly home to Perth on 25.11.99. I'm really missing home.

24.11.99

I feel even stronger again today! I'm moving better and quicker as well, which has been nice. Hayden looks good and is doing well but is taking heaps of anti-rejection tablets. They have said that in time that will reduce. It's really nice seeing him look better. He is still on painkillers and has a catheter but is moving around now and can even go outside for some fresh air. His appetite is also good. I'm still bloated though it's not as bad and haven't really got a good appetite, but that won't hurt me. Hayden is really thin so he should start to put on weight now.

25.11.99

I'm flying home today! I'm a bit worried about the flight from Adelaide to Perth but I'll be fine. Mum's coming home with me to help for six to eight weeks. They have suggested that I will need the help and I'm sure I will. I'm really lucky. I don't want to say goodbye to Hayden or Dad and Emma, but can't wait to see the kids and Grant. I'm feeling stronger and better every day now. I'm not so bloated and now wouldn't be mistaken for being pregnant! I'm still very tender around the wound itself and my shoulders aren't as bad, so all in all I'm on the mend.

26.11.99

I'm home! The trip wasn't too bad, a bit uncomfortable. I'm really tired, just want to sleep. I think travelling made me tired and, after we left the airport in Perth, the car trip home took about one and a half hours. It was really painful. Rough roads didn't help at all but I'm here and fine. I'm not as bloated today and my shoulders are heaps better but the wound is really tender again. Breanna made me laugh yesterday, after seeing me all she wanted to do was see the cut as she described it. She couldn't wait; once she had seen it she wasn't at all concerned. I'm glad Mum's here; I couldn't have done it on my own. All I did all day was sleep.

27.11.99

We spoke to Hayden today. He is still doing well and feels great. He keeps thanking me for my kidney; it has been so worthwhile. I would do it all again tomorrow just to see him well, it is all I ever wanted out of this for him to have his health and live the life he wants and so much loves. Without the transplant he would have to live in Adelaide for ages, years even, on dialysis before he could return to the station. One of Hayden's fears was rejection but in my eyes it was worth a shot whichever way it went. It is still early days for him but I do believe it will be fine.

16.12.99

I feel great, so strong now. I've had blood taken today at my doctor's here in town to check my creatine levels. My blood pressure was great and all seems good.

Hayden is well and out of hospital. He now goes in daily for blood test and in time he'll only have to go every second day and then weekly. When he gets to weekly visits he and Emma will go back to the station and live. Hayden will fly down each week to clinic for however long it takes. I'm so happy for him, he sounds so good on the phone.

18.12.99

All my test results are back and really good. I'm really feeling good now it's been four weeks since the transplant. I still get tired a bit and Mum is still with me helping but I'm doing really well. I'm going to start walking next month. My stomach around the scar is still tender, not painful just tender, especially if it is bumped but it is getting better every day.

August 2000

Well, it's been nine months since the transplant and I'm great. I'm running five days a week, I feel 100 %, and I'm back doing all that I did before and a bit more. Hayden is back working full time as head stockman and only said the other day he can't remember feeling this good. That is all the thanks I ever wanted just to hear that. It has been a long road for him and he has had a lot of setbacks over the time but is doing really well now. He flies down to clinic every three weeks and couldn't be happier. I wouldn't change a thing about being a donor, it's been really worthwhile. The thing that really surprised me through all this was people's comments. Some were great but some were just stupid. Here are a few that stand out the most: 'I hope he looks after your kidney.' My response was that it was mine while it was functioning within my body and once it was transplanted it became his and his only. 'Hope you've been left the family home and all for what you are doing.' My response was that I'm doing it because I want to. There is no price on it; it comes down to just wanting to help.

    I must point out that these are my feelings and views only. I kept a rough journal as I went through and by putting this all together I hope that it can help others in some way. When I went into this I thought it would be very straightforward, I'd have a tissue test and that would be it. How wrong I was!

As I have said, the tissue test result was the first metre in a 100-metre race. It was a race that I had planned to win from day one but it took time. We both won the race and to see and hear Hayden today makes it so rewarding for me and for him. He now has his health back and is doing what he likes best.

Cornea Transplant Story by Kerry Malone

I know corneas aren't as sexy as hearts, lungs and kidneys, but I get annoyed when most of the media attention on transplants is on these organs. Cornea transplants are not usually life saving but they are life changing. I had cornea transplants in 1990 and 1991 and this is my story.

When I was six years old I was diagnosed with cataracts. A bit unusual, as you are usually born with cataracts or have them as an older person but not normally at six years old. The first my parents knew I had a problem was when in grade 1 at school; my teacher was concerned by my squinting at the board. Off we went to see Dr Adrian Lamb and he looked after me for many years. When he retired he left me in the care of Dr Michael Walsh and during visits in the late 1980s he was telling me about cornea transplants and how he believed I was a suitable candidate for the surgery. I thought it was all a bit scary and wouldn't be in it.

In 1989 I finally gave in and said I would go to see Dr Barrett at the Lions Eye Institute at Sir Charles Gardner Hospital and hear what he had to say but no promises. The minute I met him I knew I could trust this guy with my life and before I knew it I was on the waiting list for a cornea transplant.

I was very shy and had hidden behind my glasses since I was six years old. We're talking early 1960s when I started wearing glasses and as I look at old photos I realise how lucky kids are today with the very cool frames they can choose. I call some of my glasses Dame Edna glasses because that is what they remind me of now. When I started wearing glasses they were made of glass! Mine were very thick and I still have the indents on my nose from those days. The day I tried on plastic frames was amazing! I had very thick lenses and the phrase used then was 'Coke bottle glasses', just one of the terms used to tease me throughout my schooldays.

So I am on the waiting list and thinking this will never happen. I had met a lovely guy and we had been going out for a while when we decided to go away for the weekend. We caught the boat over to Rottnest Island and were checking into the Quokka Arms, when the receptionist said she had a message for me. My sister had phoned to say Dr Barrett had called. I phoned him and he said that a suitable donor had been found. Oh my God! This was actually going to happen. I told him where I was and asked should I catch the next boat back. He said to stay and enjoy my weekend but to be at the hospital on Monday morning. I phoned my sister and my mum and then Peter did what every supportive boyfriend should do – took me to the bar at the Quokka Arms and ordered lots of alcohol!

My surgery went really well and my recovery was brilliant. I can still remember my mum driving me home from the hospital and I was wearing 'normal' sunglasses and I could see! I could read number plates of the cars in front of us! That was just with one eye done! Imagine what it would be like when they were both done. Dr Barrett was very happy with my progress and within months I was back on the waiting list for the second one.

I remember the counsellors in hospital asking how I felt about my surgery being possible through organ donation and I have been asked this question a lot over the years and my response has always been, 'I will be forever grateful to the family who during one of the worst experiences in their life made a decision which enabled me to have one of the best experiences in my life.' the only way I can explain what my surgery meant in my life is 'I have two children, but my surgery was even bigger'– that's pretty big!

I walked down the aisle when I married Peter with no glasses or contact lenses but with a new cornea, just one so I still couldn't see really well but enough to see him waiting at the end for me! My first trip to the beach by myself was a major event – all my life I had never been able to do that. I could see my towel when I came out of the water and could see other swimmers in the water with me. Likewise the first trip to the local pool and I could see the other end. I didn't have to worry about the hot water tap in the shower when I was on holidays, I could see which bottle was shampoo and which was conditioner without having to make sure I knew before I got in. I could put on some eye makeup for the first time by myself. These may sound trivial but to me they were major events.

After Peter and I were married we wanted to have kids but I wanted to wait until after my second transplant. I didn't want to have a young baby and get the call to go to hospital. I rang Dr Barrett's secretary Carol every week and I'm sure they bumped me up the list to stop me calling. The second operation was very different to the first emotionally. Peter and I were married and ready to start the next era in our lives and become parents. After my surgery there was nothing to stop us, within months I was pregnant and was able to see my babies with my new eyes!

I remember being on the bus one day on my way to a regular appointment with Dr Barrett and a woman sat next to me. She was telling me she was off to the hospital to visit her daughter who was having a cornea transplant the next day and she was feeling a bit scared, as her daughter was. I asked her who the doctor was and it was Dr Barrett. I told her my story, I had both eyes done by now and I was so glad I was there to talk to her and to see the relief as she realised her daughter was in good hands and it could work out OK as it had for me.

There have been numerous conversations over the years when I had told people what had happened to me and I know I changed people's views about organ donation.

I haven't thought about my transplants for a long time – how we take them for granted when things are going well. Recently I have had some problems with one of my eyes. I have a tear on the cornea and it looks like it may have tried to detach – after all these years. I have had significant loss of sight and some major changes have happened again in my life because of this. I am not able to drive my car and even writing this story has taken a lot of time. I am very lucky to have great family and friends who have been happily filling the role of guide dogs for me, especially after dark when I am in a bit of trouble! I'm sure my doctor has been able to buy a new car with the money I have been paying him!! I have been thinking about organ donors and transplants and all the people who have their ups and downs throughout this process and I wonder if I will have to do it again.

There has been a lot of media over the last few months about organ donation and I just wanted to write my story and let you know why I think corneas are just as sexy as hearts, lungs and kidneys!

Steve's Story

People always tell me I read the paper too much! Well, I guess if I didn't read the paper this eventful day then I wouldn't be sitting here telling my story!

I was reading the *Sunday Times* in March 2003 when I came across this article regarding a lady who needed a kidney transplant. To be honest, I looked at the heading and didn't worry about reading the rest, I went straight to the sports pages on the back. After getting my daily fix of my weekly sport I returned to the start of the paper, again breezing past this article, which took up most of the page. I turned the page to be confronted with a little ad saying 'Your Kidney Wanted'. I thought this was odd but read the advert anyway; it's at that moment I went back to the story on the other page and read the whole article. I read this article four times.

From the moment I sent the email I knew I would be the one donating my kidney. From there the long process began finding out if I was a match and to make sure my brain was on the same page as my body. I met Gail early on in the proceedings; I think if I hadn't met her I would never have gone through with this. I visited her at dialysis and saw how much not only herself but what everyone with kidney disease has to endure.

It took nearly a year for all the testing and paper work to be completed and in February 2004 we underwent the surgery at Royal Perth Hospital. I must admit that the months prior to this I was getting a little edgy. Not because I wasn't sure if I wanted to go ahead, but the amount of time it was taking. Not once throughout the entire time did I ever feel that I could not go ahead with it.

The morning of the operation was quite a whirlwind with last minute interviews with *Today Tonight* and the *Sunday Times*. I went into surgery about 8 a.m. on the Monday and the only thing I remember actually inside the theatre was telling my surgeon I didn't like his taste in music! I got back to my room at approximately 3 p.m. and don't remember much from the next two days. I was released from hospital on the Thursday but was readmitted that night with an infection in my urinary tract.

Since the operation, a lot of people ask me why I did this. My only answer so far to these questions is, because I can! I still see Gail on a regular basis and to see how much her life has changed it gives me great satisfaction in what I have done.

It has now been a year since I donated my kidney to Gail. My life is back to normal on all accounts. I restarted work two weeks after the operation and went back to sport six weeks after that. I have had no ill effects. I recently got engaged to my wonderful partner who through all of this has been a tremendous support, and we are expecting our first child in April 2005.

I get asked a lot about why there was so much media attention. Believe me if it was solely up to me all of it wouldn't have taken place, but I agreed because it was a good way to get people's attention towards organ donation. Also this was the first time in Perth a living stranger-to-stranger altruistic kidney transplant has been performed. (Well, so I have been told.)

I have also been asked how much money I got from this! As I say to them, this procedure cost me money not made me money.

Andrew and Alison

Some years ago, we were having a discussion about organ transplants. I didn't really go along with the idea, believing we were interfering with God's plan for our lives and taking the control of our lives into our own hands. Asked if I would be able to deny this chance of life for one of my own children, I wasn't able to reply with any real confidence, but felt that if I had to make such a decision, that God would give me the direction and strength at the time. Following is the story of the miracles that God performed in my walk with him to bring me to the decision that we made to have my son Andrew's organs donated.

Nothing prepared me for that day in September 1999. I was enjoying a visit from my grandson Jarrett and his partner and little girl when the phone rang. I was pleasantly surprised to get a call so early in the day from my son Michael (Michael is Andrew's identical twin). That feeling soon changed to shock and horror as Michael went on to explain that he was calling from the Darwin hospital where Andrew was in intensive care. Andrew had been admitted the night before after a road accident. Michael later told me of the chance meeting with a friend who told him about the accident. (The police have not notified us to this day.)

The doctor in charge of ICU advised that I needed to get there urgently as Andrew had suffered extensive brain injuries. Hanging up the phone I prayed long and hard for Andrew's recovery. I finished my prayer asking God to keep him safe. 'You know I desperately want to be there, but you also know that I don't have the finances to fly from Adelaide to Darwin.' Trying to hold my emotions together I went into the lounge room to tell my grandson. Repeating it all made it seem so real and so hopeless, and highlighted my frustration at not being able to do anything, other than pray. I had to let my other children know, so I phoned my son Hal who also lived in Mt Barker. A couple of hours later Hal called back to say that he had contacted everyone else and to go ahead and book my flight as he and his wife Gai would pay for my ticket.

Phoning the first airline I was told that their flight had left for the day. I phoned the second one to be told the same thing. I explained the urgency of getting on the next available flight, to be told that I was entitled to a compassionate fare, 40% off normal price. 'Thank you, Lord.' A booking was made for the next day.

My daughter Jaqi phoned from Melbourne to say that she was unable to get on the same flight but that she was booked onto a direct flight through to Darwin arriving within ten minutes of my arrival. I was sitting in the departure lounge after my son Hal had dropped me off. (He had to get the car back so his wife Gai could go to work.) I was locked in with my thoughts and dreading the four hour flight where I would just be going over the horror that I expected to confront me on arrival. How would I have the strength to face seeing my son, knowing that he had been hit by a road train? Would he still be alive when I got there? Would I be able to hold him and tell him I loved him?

Feeling a tap on my shoulder I looked up to be filled with joy and relief at seeing Jaqi standing there. Boarding the plane we discovered that I was seated across the aisle from her. We were able to freely communicate and hold hands when there was no activity in the aisle. What a comfort. After take off the pilot announced our height speed etc. The passenger seated next to me said, 'Oh, he can talk. Pity he didn't announce the flight change, I was on a direct flight to Darwin from Melbourne.' This changed my idea that Jaqi had been mixed up about her flight details. How glad I was that God had rerouted a plane for us.

We arrived at ICU to find Andrew looking as if he was peacefully sleeping. The only outward appearance of anything wrong was the life-support system and his arm in plaster. I had three days with Andrew and was able to tell him how much I loved him. How much we all loved him, and about the wonderful plan that God had for his salvation.

Arriving at the hospital one morning, Andrew's dad asked about having his organs donated. Nothing was decided, as I hadn't thought about it at all, and I said I would talk it over with the rest of the family. I thought they would agree, but had to be sure that it was something that Michael would want before I even contemplated this decision.

ICU staff was all absolutely wonderful, and when the sister said, 'Allison, we have lost him', I could feel the pain and emotion in her voice. I turned from the bed and dropped my head in my hands. 'Lord, please tell me where he is.' The most glorious feeling of peace and contentment bubbled up in me like a fountain of pure joy. This assurance was nothing that could have come from this earth, it was totally supernatural. Straight from God. I then asked the staff what was required to have Andrew's organs donated. This resulted in a flurry of activity, as the life support system had been turned off. When everything was back on track we were taken to the office to complete paperwork. The person who normally dealt with this was on holidays, so that explained how no one had spoken to us about organ donation. We learnt that Andrew's organs were healthy and okay for transplanting. The doctor contacted me later that evening to let me know that the retrieval team were on their way from Brisbane.

Sadly Vivienne (another daughter) and Hal, who had driven up from Adelaide, arrived an hour after Andrew passed into eternal life. They were able to say their goodbyes, and be a tremendous support to me by handling a lot of the paper work and funeral arrangements. The only real concern I had now was how to pay for the funeral? Someone who Viv had spoken to asked if she was aware that the Northern Territory government paid funeral costs for road accident victims? Another worry just melted away. Hal has a severe back disability and knew that he could not travel the return trip by car with Viv. I was happy to give him my ticket and travel home by car, but the airline would not hear of it. When a friend phoned me, I told her of the problem. A short time later she rang to say to go into the ticketing office that all had been sorted. The ticket was transferred into Hal's name. Another problem solved.

When Viv and I left Darwin to travel home, we had to go past the place where the accident occurred. I saw the stain from the pool of blood and felt that every bit of anguish grief anger and pain that I had been protected from begin to well up within me. I can remember taking two very deep breaths and then a gentle quiet voice saying within me, 'Don't let Satan take away the joy that I have given you, don't let him take it away now or ever.' The wonderful feeling of inner peace engulfed me once more.

The continuing miracles of Andrew's passing have been many: receiving a truly beautiful letter from Julie, the mother of Jake, Andrew's liver recipient; a lovely thank you card from a lung recipient. The donor support group who sorted out some problems with the coroner's office, and the greatest thrill of all was to meet and spend a few days with Julie, John and Jake last year. Did I need to meet Jake and his family to know that we had made the right decision? No! But meeting them reinforced that it was the right thing to do for Jake and his family and the other recipients, as well as for my family and myself.

My grandchildren and most of my family are very comfortable with the idea and those who are old enough are registered organ donors.

This week I am looking forward to a memorial service that is being held in Port Augusta for recipients and donor families. I continue to praise God for all that He has supported me through.

Laura's Story

After being misdiagnosed with asthma for many years, I was finally diagnosed with primary pulmonary hypertension (end stage) on 27 February 2002. I was told that I was terminally ill and that I had two years of life at best. I was also told that a heart and double lung transplant could be my only chance of life.

As a single mother of two boys that news was particularly devastating! This was on top of news I had received earlier that month diagnosing my eldest son Michael (then aged 15) with Asperger's syndrome (a mild form of autism)! As you would understand I became very depressed and grieved for about three months before accepting my fate.

My condition deteriorated very rapidly and within five months I was on supplemental oxygen. I was flown over to Melbourne for assessment for possible transplantation and in September 2002 I was lucky enough to be listed straight away. In fact, after my transplant one of my doctors said that when I came for assessment, one hot day could have finished me off! Arrangements were made for me to move to Melbourne to wait for my transplant, which of course meant that I had to leave my boys behind with their father. My father, Peter Perryman, came to live in Melbourne with me as my full time carer. Meanwhile my mum, Valerie, was as also left behind. Dad and I ended up living in Melbourne for nine months! Fortunately we had friends in Melbourne, enabling Mum and Dad to travel back and forth to see each other. It must have been so hard for them.

To cut a long story short, I received my transplant on 31 March 2003, and Dad and I returned home three months later, once the doctors were happy with my condition. When I woke from my transplant I had a whole new respect and appreciation for life. Prior to transplantation, Dad and I had many conversations discussing life regrets… Since I have been back home I have fulfilled many of those regrets. One of my regrets was not having a man in my life who loved and cared for me as much as I loved and cared for him. I visited a couple of online dating services in the hope to get out on the dating scene, make some new friends and hopefully find the man of my dreams.

After five months of going on dates I finally met Steve! Our first contact was on 15 August 2004 via email on RSVP.com.au, followed by many phone calls. We were supposed to have our first face-to-face date on 28th August but we couldn't wait! I told Steve that I was going into hospital for a procedure on 24 August at the Royal Adelaide Hospital (RAH) and that it would be great if he could come and visit me! He appeared at my bedside with a single long stem red rose. Dressed in my pink satin pyjamas with love hearts all over them, we walked down to a TV room where we spent the next five hours! Our relationship progressed quite quickly and by Christmas Day we were engaged!

Of course I had to put Steve through a few 'tests' before totally committing to him… Whilst I had been quite fit and healthy for some time prior to our first meeting, while participating in the Adelaide Transplant Games in September it became evident that I was becoming more and more short of breath. My health started to decline quite rapidly and I spent half my time at the RAH. During my stays in hospital Steve visited me daily and was a great source of comfort, support and happiness.

I was sent home from hospital three weeks later but was back at the RAH within a week! The doctors decided that I must have been allergic to my anti-rejection medication. After a couple of weeks adjusting my medication, despite the fact that I still wasn't feeling well, the doctors believed that my condition had stabilised and I was sent home again. On Valentine's Day 2005 I was readmitted to the RAH completely exhausted. Two days later I went into respiratory failure and ended up in intensive care. I was put in an induced coma to help me breathe and Steve was told that I had less than 40% chance of surviving. He endured this for five days until I finally awoke.

I guessed that Steve had more than passed all my tests and must truly love me to stick with me through all this! With this in mind, one of the first things I said to him when I woke up was 'So, when are we getting married?' and the rest, as they say, is history!

Margaret Pratt's Story

In 1993 I was diagnosed, after a long and difficult series of tests and explorations, with a condition called primary pulmonary hypertension, a rare condition affecting the blood vessels of the lungs whereby they become very narrow restricting blood flow to the heart. Eventually this condition leads to heart failure and ultimately death. It has no known cause and mainly affects women in their 20s and 30s. In 1993 the only treatment – not cure – for PPH was a double lung transplant.

I was a fit, healthy 33-year-old. I had a bright and exciting future and this all came crashing down around me as I sat in the doctor's office and he told me of my poor prognosis and my need for a double lung transplant. At the young age of 33, I was placed on the waiting list at the Alfred Hospital in Melbourne for a double lung transplant. My health deteriorated and I went from an independent young woman to being in a wheelchair and needing 24-hour round the clock care. I had many hospital admissions due to complications arising from my illness. I had become an exhausted shadow of myself. During this time I had to remain focused and determined to stay alive to reach transplantation. Unfortunately one in five people waiting for a transplant die before organs become available. I waited seven months before donor lungs became available.

After a 10-hour operation, one week in a coma and three more weeks in hospital recovering and learning to walk again, I left ready to restart life with the perseverance and determination that this challenge was not going to overcome me.

As I got on with my life, I began to reflect on the need to do something to support the Alfred Hospital. Of course the issue of organ rejection was on my mind. Chronic lung rejection is the most serious problem facing all lung transplant recipients and is the largest cause of death. In 2001 I was diagnosed with chronic lung rejection. By December of that year there was nothing more that could be done for me. The fear that I faced at that time was overwhelming. As I lay dying, a decision was made by the medical team to put me on the list for a second transplant. This decision was not taken lightly and the ethical and moral as well as medical implications were discussed at great length.

In January 2002 donor lungs became available and I became the first adult in Australia to undergo two successful double lung transplants.

The Margaret Pratt Foundation is currently supporting a project at the Alfred looking into treating rejection with a combination of drugs. You can appreciate that this will take a lot of time and results will not happen overnight.

The cost of keeping this research going over the next three years is about $200,000 and the Margaret Pratt Foundation needs your help to raise this money. While the overall value of this research will benefit lung transplant recipients it will potentially influence the management of other organ transplant recipients as well as the care of other conditions such as asthma and bronchitis.

My life expectancy is uncertain, but I am continuing to work hard to raise money for research into lung transplantation.

Many lung transplants are not successful in the long term. Ninety per cent of recipients survive beyond 12 months. However, this figure drops to 50% after five years. The Margaret Pratt Foundation aims to improve these figures.

Living Kidney Donor Story – Sue & Vic

♥

My stepdaughter Sue had been diagnosed with renal problems at age 18, and at 24 began dialysis for the next five years. She worked full time for the Red Cross for four years of her dialysis period but due to her declining health changed to part time work for the last year of dialysis so she could have treatment during the day on her non-work days instead of after work. The Red Cross was wonderfully supportive and understanding of her condition and Sue is still working there today.

When my wife Carol and I visited Sue at the dialysis unit, I always felt sad for Sue and the other patients who had no choice but to undertake this procedure three times a week if they wanted to survive. As well as dialysis, there are regular clinic check up visits and other medical procedures to face from time to time including operations for new fistulas, the insertion point for dialysis needles when the other fails.

There is also the daily assortment of medications to take, and various other health issues which can occur for this condition. I was always extremely humbled by Sue's unselfish, uncomplaining nature and her courage, despite the handicap she had endured for so long. There is a long waiting list for donor kidneys and one person in Australia dies every week waiting (source: Kidney Health Australia).

Due to the long period on dialysis, Sue's treatment was not working as effectively any more and her health was deteriorating. Without Sue's knowledge, I asked to be tested for my suitability as a living donor. As is required by medical ethics, I was referred to an independent nephrologist who explained what was involved.

I underwent a series of tests over the next six months until they were reasonably sure that I was a compatible donor. Sue was then informed about the possibility of a transplant and was overwhelmed by the news. Further tests for both of us then ensued and a period of anxiety followed while we waited for the final test results, which were OK. All systems go!

Our operations were performed on 25 November 2002 at Royal Perth Hospital and were successful with no problems. I was discharged three days later, and Sue about a week after that. I would like to pay tribute to all the hospital and clinic staff in all the various fields for their support, care and skills in giving kidney patients a better life. These wonderful people go largely unheralded for their dedication and for the lives they save. Thank you!

In November 2003, at age 30, Sue was married to her long-time supportive partner Justin and to see them both so radiant and happy on their wedding day made it all worthwhile. I still feel elated seeing the difference it has made to the quality of Sue's life. My wish for Sue and Justin is that they have many happy years ahead of them. I have absolutely no regrets at my decision to donate. It is the most rewarding thing I have ever done in my life.

The Gift of Life – An Organ Donor Saved My Life

♥

In 1992 I was diagnosed with a kidney disease called IgA nephropathy. By August 1994, my condition had deteriorated to end stage renal failure and I had commenced haemodialysis.

On the Easter weekend of 1995, I went for my first holiday where I would dialyse away from my home-treating hospital. I was staying at the Galilee Holiday flats at a secluded location called Nungurner in East Gippsland, without any phone connected. Although I had borrowed a mobile phone (the size of a brick!) for the weekend, it didn't work. I was on the transplant waiting list and effectively I was uncontactable. I had dialysis at the Latrobe Regional Hospital on the Saturday and I clearly recall the nurse saying to me, 'Sadly, Easter is a time when there are accidents on the road and organs become available.'

Just two days later, on Monday 17 April, after having a kick of a footy with friends, we headed back to our holiday flat to discuss options for lunch. We agreed to take the boat to the Metung pub for a counter lunch. Moments before setting off, my girlfriend's mother suggested we should pop the cork from a bottle of champagne. It seemed strange to have a bottle of champagne before going out for lunch but we didn't complain!

Still enjoying the champagne, eyebrows were raised at the appearance of a police divvy van (paddy wagon) at our remote and tranquil location. Heading in our direction, the police asked if I was among the throng. By this stage I was having heart palpitations and, in the back of my mind, I was hoping for a miracle. The officer asked me how long I intended to stay on holiday and I told him, 'As long as I can – unless I get a better offer!' He then broke the amazing news that the hospital had a kidney for me and needed me there as soon as possible.

It was nearly 1 p.m. and I needed to be in Melbourne by 5 p.m. And it was Easter Monday – the roads would be chaos! But the police were on hand to take charge of the situation. They drove my girlfriend and me to Bairnsdale airfield. Police divvy vans, for the uninitiated, are basically a tin box with seat belts – but boy, do they move! At Bairnsdale we boarded an Air Ambulance helicopter for a special, and at times turbulent, journey to Royal Park.

At the Royal Melbourne Hospital I had a blood transfusion and dialysed for the last time. Later that night I was wheeled down the corridor to the operating theatre, a small, battered polystyrene esky balanced on my lap. Within that esky was not, as you might ordinarily expect, a six-pack of beer. Instead, that esky contained the ultimate gift that words can't even begin to describe. It was my gift of life.

I woke up plugged into a myriad of tubes and machines. It was a new beginning. The operation was a success and I was well enough to leave the hospital a week later. I later found out that with 5.6 antigens, only a twin brother could have provided me with a better-matched kidney.

Thankfully on that Easter Monday my mother had decided to drop in to my house to do some ironing while I was away, so she took the initial call from the hospital. It seems fitting that the one to give me life took the call that ultimately saved my life. My mother immediately called my sister, who in turn called the police for help with the situation. Fortunately the police were able to assist – above and beyond the call of duty!

The final twist in the story – the champagne. If we hadn't popped the cork on that bottle before heading to lunch, we would have been out in the boat and the police would have had no option but to advise the hospital that they couldn't contact me. The kidney would no doubt have gone to an equally appreciative and grateful recipient, however I can't be sure I would be here today. I still have that bottle – empty of champagne but full of meaning. It has pride of place in my wall unit at home.

And to the moral of the story… This life changing event, and the very fact that I am still here to talk about it, would not have happened without the consent of a very special person to organ donation. This most generous gift of life has enabled me to enjoy a healthy, active lifestyle. To my donor family, I am and always will be deeply and eternally grateful. In January this year I wrote to thank my donor's family and recently received a beautiful reply. I intend to remain in contact with my donor mother long into the future. To the people who played the various important roles involved in organ donation and transplantation – from the organ donation coordinators, the police and ambulance officers, to the surgeons, nurses and social workers – I am here because of you. It may just be 'all in a day's work' for these professionals, but 10 years on their 'day's work' has had a wonderful, lasting impact on my life. I appreciate that work now every bit as much as I did then.

In this, the 10-year anniversary of my transplant, I want to do my bit to raise awareness of the importance of organ donation by sharing my story with you. By raising the profile of and awareness about the critical nature of organ donation, I am hopeful that waiting lists will become a thing of the past. With only one quarter of Australia's population currently listed on the Australian Organ Donor Register, there is great potential to significantly increase the number of names on the register. It is interesting to note that among Western nations, Australia has a comparatively low rate of organ donation, yet a very high rate of transplant success. Bridging the gap between the two is the primary challenge.

Are YOU an organ donor?

WOW! - Lisa Upton's Story

Organ donation and transplants are things I had never really thought about. Now I know how important they are, because without the amazing generosity of my donor family I would not be enjoying my life today. After months of doctor's visits and my condition getting worse, I was told that my only option was a double lung transplant.

The day I got the call to say they found a match for me, was the best and the most frightening day of my life. It's now been two years since my transplant (Australia Day 2004) and I still have to pinch myself to believe it really happened. But I didn't think that day would come, as time was running out. I had been on oxygen 24/7 and it had taken me a good 12 months to finally have the courage to say yes to the transplant. I don't know why, maybe I thought I would get better. The odds of me surviving the operation weren't in my favour either but, having a wonderful husband and two boys, I knew I had to fight and take the chance.

My life, you could say, has been very eventful. At the age of two I was diagnosed with a Wilms tumour, which affected my lungs, kidneys and stomach. After years of chemotherapy and radiation, my poor body had taken a battering. With great parents and an older brother behind me I managed to live a very good childhood. Due to the radiation that I had on my lungs for the cancer, I suffered pulmonary fibrosis, which scarred my lungs and restricted my breathing and also made me get tired and puffed very easy, but that didn't stop me doing normal things; I just knew my limits.

Later in my life I married a wonderful man and we decided to have a family. Doctors told us there could be complications and I may not be able to have kids. We decided to try and we now have two wonderful boys. I then started to get more tired and puffed out. So that was the reason for the doctors' visit.

Having finally agreed to go ahead with the transplant, the day I got the call to say they found a match was a bit of a blur. Being from South Australia I had to go to the Alfred Hospital in Melbourne for the operation. Watching my two boys, family and friends faces out of the Royal Flying Doctor plane window was very hard and emotional with the thought that I might never see them again. I had to stay in Melbourne for about three months before I could return home to SA. That was also hard because it was a long time to be away from family and friends.

After spending about three weeks in ICU, then moving to a normal ward, my husband returned home to bring our boys over to Melbourne to be with us as a family while I recovered. Once I started rehabilitation, walking around with my kids was fantastic. Then after returning home, walking them to school, wow, what a great feeling that was.

Transplant was a very scary word at the time. Thinking, how could they take out my lungs and replace them with someone else's, and also the thought that someone had to die first. To me organ donors are like angels. Now two years on, I'm still amazed at how I'm breathing and living a wonderful life with my family. Having a second chance at life is, to me, very special.

My Story – Bob Pocock

I began smoking at the age of about 13. No real reason apart from that it was the cool thing to do. No one mentioned any dangers related to smoking, at least not then. The year would have been 1961 or thereabouts, so when my story really starts I would have been 48 years old.

I was first diagnosed with pneumonia in August of 1996 and was put on the normal antibiotics by the GP, but the condition never got any better. After a few months, it was pretty evident that something else was seriously wrong. I asked the GP if I could see a specialist, and finally came into contact with a great Doctor who knew what was wrong. He diagnosed me with COAD (chronic obstructive airways disease) or emphysema as it is more commonly called. I then went through a series of tests that took forever at the RAH, and the outcome was not good.

Such things as lung reduction and lung transplant were discussed, but I really can't recall much of what was being said. Luckily my wife understood what was what, as I was dumbstruck. I was finally told that my only option was a lung transplant. Depending on my state of health I would go through another series of tests both here in Adelaide and in Melbourne and hopefully be accepted on the waiting list for a transplant. After another few months I was put on that list in December 1997.

The next few months would be hell on earth for both my wife and myself. Eventually I ended up in a wheelchair, as I didn't have the breath to walk even the shortest distance. Waiting for the call that may or may not come was really weighing heavily on both of us.

By July of 1998, my condition had deteriorated so much that I was on oxygen for 20 hours daily, and was virtually house bound.

After a false alarm on 7 September and flying all the way to Melbourne, only to be told that the donor organ was no good and turned back home, the real thing happened on 25 September. I was taken by ambulance to Adelaide airport, then by Air Ambulance to Melbourne and then by ambulance to the Alfred Hospital. I was operated on in the early hours of 26 September. Everything went well, thankfully.

I had to remain in Melbourne for my recovery period of three months, with my carer (who happens to be my lovely wife), and live on a budget. No promises or guarantees were given, but here it is two years later and no oxygen, no puffers, no nebuliser but a lot of medication.

I have nothing but praise and admiration for the staff at the Alfred. My thanks to everyone – Dr Julian Smith (surgeon), Louise McFarlane, Anne Griffiths, Wendy, the physios, and especially the great nursing staff at 5D. Without their dedication, care and attention, and outlook, I am quite sure some of us would never have made it.

2001

Who would have thought three years ago that I would still be here today. Just turned 53 years old and still feeling great. Still playing ten-pin bowling and enjoying life to the fullest. In February 2002 another grandchild by my son and his wife. That makes five grandchildren in all. I am now an active member of Transplant SA and am currently helping two others from Lyell McEwin and one from RAH who are in the same predicament that I was in four years ago. I'm thankful that I can be of some help and comfort to these people. I know what it was like when Mary and I had no one to confide in.

2003

Quite a lot has happened to me over the last two years but none as noteworthy as late 2002 and early 2003. I returned to full-time study in August 2002 to gain my Certificate III Support Worker, Disability. In February 2003 I began work with Leveda. This is a company that manages 13 houses in the general community that house people with severe physical disabilities and two houses with intellectually disabled persons. I have worked in more than one of these houses over the last nine months and I have enjoyed it immensely. Then in November I began working for PQA as well and I now have a permanent client for five hours every Friday. Again, a position I enjoy immensely.

Another few years have passed and it's now January 2006. Still going strong even after a heart attack last March. A few more medications but it's no big deal. Still working but now for four agencies, both with Disability and Aged Care, and still doing some study to complete my Certificate IV.

I still have to take a lot of medication, have three-monthly check-ups at the Royal Adelaide Hospital for my transplant, and other check-ups on a regular basis for other minor problems but they are less and less of a bother than they were in the beginning. I have met a lot of other transplant recipients who have had not only lung transplants, but kidney, pancreas, heart, heart and lung and a number of other different organs. We all have one thing in common – we are grateful for the unselfish act of giving a transplant organ and we are all one of a kind in a very select, elite group.

Dylan's Story 18.3.1993-23.10.2005

♥

Dylan was born on a hot Saturday 18 December at 5.40 p.m. – a healthy six-pound two-ounce baby boy. Slightly jaundiced, he required a blood transfusion and oxygen, nothing too bad, as no one told me any different.

1995

While Dylan was in hospital with a bout of rotavirus, the doctors mentioned he might have asthma. One of the nurses at the hospital had a chat with me and suggested I talk with the paediatrician as she felt there was something more. She had been keeping a very close eye on him but she didn't want to alarm us. She said the doctors do their job, but we are with the children day and night and we get to see and monitor them closely. We went for a follow-up appointment with the paediatrician. He listened to Dylan's heart then said it might be worth an appointment with a specialist so we could get a clearer understanding if there was something there or not. Later, he told us he suspected a heart murmur.

Friday 27 February we went to see a paediatric cardiologist at the old children's hospital in Camperdown. After doing an ultrasound he could tell us Dylan had an ASD (arial septrim defect) that would probably need repairing when he was about five years old. He said there was high pressure in his lungs but it might be due to ASD. He wanted to see us in 12 months for review. So we went home and didn't worry.

1996

We went to see a paediatric cardiologist again, this time at Westmead, and he said that ASD closure would be done sooner rather than later as he was concerned about the pressure.

Dylan was admitted to hospital in June with difficulty breathing. He was put on Ventolin and Tilade. The paediatrician said it was asthma-like symptoms due to bronchitis. In July we went to see the surgeon who was performing Dylan's operation and he was very helpful with our questions and concerns and we were put on a waiting list. The only thing we found extremely hard was to sign the paper in case something happened during the surgery, but we understood why.

One Saturday night, we were sitting at home watching *Hey Hey It's Saturday* and the phone rang. It was the Children's Hospital at Westmead asking us to bring Dylan in the next day for surgery on Monday morning. It all happened so fast my head was spinning and Ayman went into shutdown. I was up half the night packing and just couldn't sleep.

Ayman carried him down to theatre and I waited outside for him to come out. He went to get the paper and I went for a cup of tea. It's such a trying time when your child, let alone your only child, is somewhere you have no control over whatsoever. But these men and women are professional in their field and we do trust them, we have to. During his time in surgery I didn't know what to do, Narelle came over from university and that passed a couple of hours. I was so happy to see her, I had held together until I started making her a cup of tea and was talking about the operation and I just broke down, but boy what a relief.

At last, after four hours in surgery, he was in recovery and we were allowed to see him. He stayed in ICU overnight. The pressure in his lungs was still high and his heart was slightly enlarged. He was moved back to the ward the next morning.

Dylan had a lung scan that showed he had some blood clots and the paediatric cardiologist wanted to talk to us about the operation. He said Dylan had a rare disease called pulmonary hypertension. It is progressive narrowing of the blood vessels of the lungs causing high blood pressure in these vessels and eventually leads to heart failure. The doctor thought by bringing his ASD closure forward it might help. He said this is a very rare disease of unknown cause, we will keep a good eye on him but he was also concerned about the blood clots. When we went home he was on two litres of oxygen 24-hourly, Digitoxin, Intel and Warfarin and was to see the paediatric cardiologist in January.

Overall, Dylan appeared well and as active as he could be, and the PH never stopped him from being a normal, naughty, loveable little boy.

1997

To be taken off oxygen is a godsend. It limited the things we could do with such big tanks, as we didn't have little portable ones. Dylan had a blood test and lung perfusion scan. The scan showed no change since the last one in November 1996. The paediatric cardiologist spoke of possibly taking him off Warfarin for a period.

In April Dylan had a cardiac catheterisation to see if nitric oxide may help the pressure. Again the doctor warned us of the risks involved. At this stage we were hoping for a miracle. He didn't come out of the anaesthesia well, and had a very high temperature, so we stayed overnight as I didn't feel comfortable taking him home. The following day he was fine. He will stay off the Warfarin and have oxygen at night. Dylan also started having the flu vaccine every year as a precaution.

In October he went in for a sleep study. He found that a bit scary, with all the wires and glue on his head. It ended up being a very restless night for him; he wasn't very well and they said they would have to repeat it again at a later date.

His fourth birthday was celebrated at McDonalds, again a fun time had by all, and we made an elephant cake to take in for preschool, he loved the elephants.

1998

Throughout the year he continued speech therapy and improved well. He also kept on with the swimming, his teacher was great and Dylan really liked her.

Dylan was reviewed in May by the paediatric cardiologist, the first time since his operation in September. The PH was persistent and due to his desaturation at night they left the oxygen on at night. At this stage he has no cardiac related symptoms. He weighed 15 kilograms. There was a slight right ventricular over activity and a slapping second heart sound with no murmurs as before. We had an oximeter delivered from the hospital to read his saturations for a couple of nights to see what was happening. I can still remember the bell going off half the night.

Echocardiography showed mild right ventricular hypertrophy, but perhaps a little less right ventricular dilation, and a somewhat more normalised left ventricular configuration than at his last visit. There was no tricuspid incompetence, preventing assessment of the right ventricular pressure, and the main pulmonary artery remains dilated.

We spoke to the doctor about our forthcoming trip to Fiji in June. He said the oxygen could be difficult, so Dylan was able to be off it while we were away. He is also booked in for another lung perfusion. The doctor will see him in six months.

July saw Dylan back at the Children's Hospital for a sleep study. He remembered what happened before, but bribery is a wonderful tool to a parent in time of need, even as little as an ice cream. He did well and if he sat still they could use plaster instead of glue, which is a lot easier to get out. There was nothing significant in their findings. They found that the oxygen helped his saturations keep to at least 95%.

1999

We will see the paediatric cardiologist before Dylan starts school. He will outline for the school what Dylan has and present a plan of attack if anything was to occur. Dylan continues to have clear evidence of modest pulmonary hypertension but this seems to be stable and well tolerated. He continued his oxygen at night and we talked about strategies for selection of sports over the next few years – no contact sport, running or squads. Golf or chess – Dylan was not impressed.

Dylan started school in February, all happy and didn't cry until two weeks in. About the third week after he started he was in hospital for two weeks with pneumonia. Pneumonia was something he got frequently. He made sure his school work kept up to date; that's one thing he didn't like to fall behind in. He continued his swimming lessons and speech therapy. I helped out in the tuck shop and with reading groups. It was a sneaky way to get to be with him a little without him noticing.

We saw the paediatric cardiologist in May and Dylan is to continue his oxygen at ¼-litre at night. He is well after his episode of pneumonia. There are no signs of heart failure. There was mild precordial overactivity with a loud second and a puffing systolic murmur at the right sternal edge. His cardiac findings remain stable, with features of moderate pulmonary hypertension, which seems well tolerated. No new recommendations and will visit again in six months.

Dylan's first disco at school was in June. He was always a stylish boy (something he got from his dad), he was all ready and he had the best time while I was in a corner somewhere with his oxygen in tow, in floods of tears just to see him so full of life and having fun, something others often take for granted.

He didn't really participate in sports days but I think he may have realised there were going to be things that his body wouldn't allow him to do. He never got down about not being able to do sports like that, or took it out on the other children; he just got on with it. July brought around a different kind of sport that Dylan might be able to play – T-ball. We went down to sign up and we had a bit of a hit and he enjoyed it. He trained Thursday afternoons after school and played on a Saturday morning for about 1½ hours. He was a good little hitter and catcher. It was really good to see him be part of a team and have fun. I think he enjoyed it too as Ayman was manager and helped out with training, it was great for them both.

In November both of us were baptised together. I will never forget that closeness we shared. It was a very special moment.

2000

Back to school year 1, swimming, T-ball, but no more speech therapy. I asked him if he wanted to learn music and he said he would like to learn guitar.

That year was a rocky road for all of us. Ayman and I separated in February for 10 months but were able to sort things out and reunited in November. It was hard for Dylan and being so young he didn't fully understand, but we both knew how important it was that he knew we both loved him as much as ever.

In March, year 1 went to the zoo for an excursion. Dylan had a good time but his teacher was concerned about how breathless he got and found it hard to keep up to the others. I don't really think I had been witness to him being tired and breathless.

In April we went to the Royal Easter Show and thoroughly enjoyed it, all the animals and the show bags. It tired him out immensely but he still wanted to go. Last time we went he was in the pram.

In August Dylan had an appointment with the specialist from the sleep study unit. We went to the Sleep Disorder Centre in Annandale. He spoke to Dylan and me about how Dylan was going. He was a very nice doctor, you don't usually see him when you have your sleep study at the hospital. The study starts late about 8 p.m. and finishes at 5 a.m. and the nurses take care of everything. He was lovely with Dylan, and funny. Dylan liked him as he did his other doctors and nurses that cared for him.

Dylan had another sleep study in November. His saturation was studied in room air for two hours in non-REM sleep and remained between 94% and 98%. However, in REM sleep, physiological pauses resulted in mild drops in oxygen saturation to a minimum level of 91%. The supplemented oxygen reversed these changes. He was to stay on oxygen at night and have a clinical review in six months, and a sleep study in one year's time.

Presentation day was in December and the teacher said to me, 'If you can try to get here that would be great.' Well, I was sure we could. Dylan received a Merit Certificate for Citizenship: Positive and Caring Attitude. We were so proud of him, of course I was crying.

2001

Going into a year 1/2 composite class showed us that Dylan could work independently. He has continued all his activities. His health has remained stable. He is currently taking Warfarin and Nifedipine, Ventolin and Flixotide.

He had a follow-up appointment with the paediatric cardiologist, who suggested we try him on 24-hourly oxygen again to see if that might help the pressure, and also help at school. It was remarkable how he handled that time. He was very nervous at first as the children would stare and ask questions but we talked about it and I spoke to his class and in the end if anyone asked he simply said, 'The oxygen helps my lungs.' That year was the only time he didn't have pneumonia. He took it on board and dealt with it whichever way he knew how.

In April we received an email from our friend, who lives in the United States, with the name of a Hospital that specialises in PH. After email back and forth our paediatric cardiologist informed us that he was involved in studies worldwide in PH, that many of the overseas centres claim 'expertise' in this area, but much of the data is pooled and well known to relevant clinicians. He is going to Toronto, Paris and Germany where he will meet up with most of the world experts in PH. But he encouraged us to keep exploring and comparing notes.

In May Dylan was admitted to Edgar Stephen ward for an increase of the Nifedipine and a holter monitor for 24 hours. He was booked in for a sleep study that night as well.

A review with the paediatric cardiologist showed that the PH had increased over the last 12 months. It's so hard to believe when you think his pressure must be going down because he seems so well. He didn't respond to the Nifedipine. His heart rate is good and the plan is to increase the tablet again. The cardiologist plans to see him December, and if the situation remains the same he will reduce the daytime oxygen to establish whether this alters the degree of PH and early next year consider other experimental oral agents available in trial use for PH, including Sildenafil.

I enjoyed going up to school and helping after work and seeing him with his friends. Dylan loved school; it was the only normal part of his life. He went on the walk-a-thon with his oxygen in the trolley. I wheeled it for him but I think he did three or four laps of the school. He had done well. Also in May he went to a skate plus night for a fundraiser for school and I noticed he was getting tired quickly. He would come off and have a sit and a bit of oxygen and off he would go again.

In October he was on Warfarin and nifedipine but the Nifedipine didn't show any evidence of doing anything. Throughout this his saturations stayed good (95%). He had a cardiac catheterisation done but little response to either oxygen or nitric oxide. He was also on Adalat for a while. Our cardiologist spoke to the guys in Melbourne and they suggested trying Bosentan. He said we'd try the Adalat for a while and keep the Bosentan in mind.

2002

Year 3 and in primary school. He didn't stay on Adalat for too long; they stopped that and started him on a calcium blocker, Cardizem. He doesn't have his oxygen all the time, just at night, which he is over the moon about. He sat the basic skills test and did very well; he never fell behind in his schoolwork.

Dylan is still doing T-ball but has now upgraded to the next level, which is Soft Toss. He has had enough of swimming, so now he can concentrate on Soft Toss and his guitar. I would rather him enjoy what he does instead of being too tired.

One sunny morning in March, Dylan was out the front riding his scooter when he fell off it and broke his arm – the same arm as the trampoline episode. He really thought that was cool with his bright green plaster. As he was left handed, he didn't think he had to do any work. 'Don't think you'll get out of work that easy,' I told him. Sure enough, we improvised and he was able to do a lot of work on the computer.

Not long after that he became unwell at school and was sent to the hospital by ambulance, as the colour apparently just drained from him. His teacher went with him and he told the ambulance officer he was feeling off due to his paediatrician giving him an overdose of Fluvax. The doctor came to see him later and couldn't believe what Dylan had said. 'I thought you were my friend,' I remember him saying. Dylan was very serious about the matter; it was funny how he made his own diagnosis. He stayed overnight and went home the next afternoon.

In April he had another ECG holter attached for the night. In May he had a cardiac catheterisation and angiogram done at the Children's Hospital, but there was little response to either oxygen or nitric oxide. Review with Doctor in two months.

When we saw the paediatric cardiologist in July, we discussed the trial drug Bosentan and decided to go ahead as there was a lot of paper work involved. In August it was approved, so Dylan will be admitted to the Children's Hospital to start in September. Like a lot of drugs, it has side effects, but with something like PH your options are minimal. He already has a lot of blood tests due to being on Warfarin so hopefully they can do a liver function test at the same time. There may be future fertility impairment. We hope and pray if he gets to that age where all that is relevant, then we will explain but for now all we can do is think about today and keeping him here with us a little longer.

We went down to Skate Plus in November but he found it very tiring and this time he sat down most of the time. I think that was the last time we went, and he loved it so much.

2003

Back to see the paediatric cardiologist. Dylan's liver function tests (LFT) have all been normal. The ultrasound had a slight increase in the pressure. If the LFT stays normal he will consider increasing the night-time dose. Overall things seem relatively stable. Review in two months. Also in January our dentist wanted an orthodontist to have a look at Dylan, as if he hasn't enough to cope with. He has severe crowding.

In April we went to Blue Gum Farm with Fran and Sammy and again they had a great time. They had a running race and I thought that would be the end of Dylan, I don't even know what made him do it, but he did and he wasn't too bad after it. It was hard a lot of the time watching him stand back, but he knew his limits and how he felt if he pushed too much. As a child it must have been so frustrating for him.

In early August Dylan became unwell at school, so I made arrangements to take him to see his paediatrician. We were there for a very long time and had to go to the children's ward to have blood tests done. Dylan was very tired by this stage. He also had an X-ray and ultra sound. He ended up having viral pneumonia and influenza.

In September Dylan was unwell during the night so I rang the registrar on call at the Children's Hospital and he suggested we go over in the morning for an ultrasound. He was so sick, he could hardly walk. He was coughing, and I don't think we had seen him so unwell. He had viral pneumonia and influenza. After waiting in emergency for hours we went up to Edgar Stephen Ward (he called it his ward) he was on IV antibiotics for a week and they had to increase his oxygen to four litres to get it back up to 95%.

They had to take blood tests daily, ultrasounds and chest X-rays, and he just wanted to be left alone. During his stay, the cardiologist spoke with me and said to prepare ourselves for the worst. I thought, 'No way, he'll come good', and sure enough he came good, but it took a lot out of him. I don't really think he recovered from that. Irreversible damage had been done to his heart and lungs, even though he was a little fighter this really set him back. He was in hospital for eight days and went home on Augmentin, Flixotide, Ventolin, Bosentan and Cardizem. Dylan will see the Paediatrician next week and the paediatric cardiologist in four weeks.

I started seeing a lovely social worker from the hospital during that visit in hospital. Dealing with the unknown of PH is bad enough, let alone all the other stuff that goes with it. Even Dylan dealing with his anger is very sad, and not knowing which way is the best way to try and help him. At one stage Dylan became both physically and verbally abusive towards me, and I just didn't know what to do. I realise he had to let it out but I didn't want to be always in the firing line. The social worker and I thought maybe we could get together with Dylan and talk about a few things. I couldn't believe my child could be so blunt, and I thought rude, but she assured me later it was OK. 'Why should I talk to you about my personal business?' he asked. I could feel that I was going to cop it when we left, and I did. The social worker said to me he was being assertive and she felt that it was OK for him to want to keep things private and not want strangers to know everything about him. He had a choice to share and he chose not to. That was such a rough patch; it felt like he was a rebellious teenager.

One day we were off to the doctors and we had a good chat about what he wanted as far as when we would visit the doctors. 'I'm sick of having to be sent out of the room so you can talk about me,' he said. 'Well, what can you do about it, Dylan,' I said to him. We got over to Westmead to see the paediatric cardiologist and we went in and after checking Dylan's height and weight, he asked Dylan could he speak to Mum and Dad, and could he wait outside. Well, he took a big breath and said, 'Do you mind if stay?' and the doctor said, 'Of course you can.'

We bought an oximeter to read his saturations at home and the school had a fundraiser to raise money to help with its upkeep. We went to the cathedral in the city a few times and two ladies, plus his scripture teacher, were specifically praying for his Jesus to heal Dylan's heart and lungs. He cried and cried; it was overwhelming, especially when he prayed and asked for healing himself. He has a true faith and knows that there are so many people everywhere praying for him and that helps us get through the tough times.

2004

In March, Ayman and I went down to Melbourne, without Dylan, to meet the medical team that specialises in PH in children. We spoke about the drug Sildenafil, which can be used with Bosentan. We had a good chat with the specialist and he offered us a medicine called Prostacyclin (Flolan), which is administered through a central line. We also touched on transplant; he did mention the survival rate was very poor in children; they have made a policy decision in Victoria not to do this operation before the age of 15 years. That option was a long way off as Dylan was a very slight build and would take a lot to get to the body weight requirement. It also usually adds only a few years to their life and these may be complicated by significant medical problems requiring close medical attention. We found the visit extremely worthwhile as far as other therapeutic options.

In July Dylan went into the Children's Hospital to start a new tablet,

Sildenafil. He was in hospital for five days and it was sort of a holiday for Dylan, as he wasn't sick, and he was able to visit the Starlight Room and play the Play Station. He got on really well with the nurses; some of them had been there since his first admission. So his tablets are Bosentan, Sildenafil, Cardizem, Warfarin, Ventolin, Flixitide and oxygen at night.

Later that month he was admitted to the Westmead Children's Hospital with a viral infection for a week. He still seems unwell even with the introduction of Sildenafil.

In May, Sammy's sister had a baby girl and Dylan loved this little baby. His face would light up whenever he saw her.

It's all getting frustrating and scary as nothing is helping him and we are running out of ideas and medicine to help. It is really hard to stand back and virtually watch your son sinking in front of your eyes. He is not responding to any medication whatsoever.

After some thinking about transplant, we came to the conclusion that we should at least get into the loop with St Vincent's Hospital. I sent a letter to Dylan's paediatric cardiologist for a referral to a transplant surgeon. He was very obliging. His condition over the last few months seems to have worsened. Even if he was to be on a list, that would be a step forward.

I had to deal with a very delicate matter at school regarding Dylan and what would happen if someone was to ask him was he going to die. One of the parents had bought this up with our principal. I took this question to our minister. We spoke of how Dylan answered very confidently and honesty when having to take the oxygen cylinder and trolley to school with him every day and thought he could continue that approach. I asked Dylan that very question. 'Dylan, if one of the children asked if you were going to die, what would you say?' His reply was 'My lungs are not real good and I get puffed out easily, but I feel well today, thanks.' I'm so glad he was direct but honest, a special trait to have.

Sport was never much of a problem for Dylan as he knew his limits, but as he grew older it took a toll on his body and as the registration of baseball was getting close he had to make a choice about signing up for the next season or not, and he chose to stand down. Such a hard call for a child but it had to be his choice. People constantly said he was an old man in a young body, that may have been so, but the choices and decisions he made were after a lot of thought; he was very rational.

During the July holidays we went to South West Rocks for a week. Dylan's illness has been extremely difficult for Ayman and it's such a joy to see them together having fun, fishing or just hanging out. Dylan wasn't well; he was really clingy with Ayman and miserable; he had no life in him.

When we got home, Dylan still wasn't very well so he went to the paediatrician and he was admitted to the Westmead Children's Hospital with a gastro bug. He still seems unwell even with the introduction of Sildenafil. I felt so bad, not realising what was wrong. He had to go through all the blood test routine again when we got home from hospital, which was horrible.

Since Dylan has had the respect of the doctors, he seems a lot more content. It had to be his call as far as asking to stay in the room because they would appreciate that if he is asking he must be ready. Even though we think he has known a lot more than we ever did about what's been going on with his body. Slowly decreasing the Bosentan; to be taken off soon.

In September Dylan went on a Starlight Escape decked out as a pirate ship. We went out on Sydney Harbour – it was great and, also in September, he was granted his Starlight Wish, which was to go to Dubbo zoo and stay overnight. We went with Dylan's friend Sammy and Fran, which was just great. We stayed at Dubbo for three nights before going to the zoo to stay overnight. Dylan's favorite animal is the elephant. He has a big collection, and he got to touch Yum Yum, his little face was priceless. We will never forget that time, it was wonderful.

In November 2004 we took Dylan down to Melbourne to visit the PH team. They ran all the usual tests on him and he is certainly struggling and getting worse. After a six-minute walk, his saturations fell from 95% to 90%. He was definitely breathless and struggled towards the end. We decided, after talking with our Cardiologist, that the IV medicine was not for Dylan and a lung transplant was not an option. He was taken off Bosentan. When we got back from Melbourne we were off to Canberra for a school excursion. Dylan went down on the bus and I followed. He got to stay in with the other kids; they didn't get much sleep by the look of them the next morning. Dylan slept on the floor, as the slats on his bed were all broken, and that was a great laugh for the boys for a while.

We met with the paediatric cardiologist in December, again without Dylan, to discuss what our next steps were. We spoke about re-introducing Bosentan as the doctors in Melbourne suggested. His clinical health was no different on the Bosentan with the Sildenafil than off so we left that as is. We had thought long and hard about lung transplant and resigned ourselves to the fact that it was not an option. As far as the Prostacyclin is concerned, it is obvious none of the other medications demonstrated benefit to him and this being a very invasive drug it just isn't an option for Dylan. The Prostacyclin is also very expensive – $150,000 to $200,000 dollars a year, which they would try to get on compassionate grounds through the Department of Health or the company; it is funded in Victoria but not here. The doctor would be more than happy to help us if we wanted to go down that road.

We noticed the change in him these last twelve months and how he has deteriorated, which is to be expected but very hard to accept that one day, because of the PH, he won't be with us any more. He's 11 years old now and we wonder what the New Year has in store for us. I try and imagine life without Dylan and I think I know what it will be like. It's very strange as a parent, and I think especially as a mum, to put yourself in that mode of thinking. It's like you step out of yourself and it's a completely different person it's happening to.

2005

We saw the cardiologist in January, before we went away on holidays, and it is very obvious that he has worsened over the last two to three years. He is currently on Sildenafil, Cardizem, Warfarin, Ventolin when needed, Flixotide and still the oxygen at night. He weighed in at 23 kilograms and 132 centimetres. The ultrasound didn't pick up anything out of the ordinary and his cardiac status remained stable. We pushed up the Sildenafil a little higher and we spoke about the usual flu vaccine before winter and the pneumococcal vaccine as well. Other than that, Dylan was happy to be going on holidays.

Towards the end of March he was complaining of a pain in the chest at school a couple of times and feeling breathless. We went to the Paediatrician but he couldn't explain it and thought it might be bad indigestion from what Dylan was telling him.

In April we set up a meeting with the Lung Transplant Unit at St Vincent's Hospital in Sydney purely to get into the loop and to let them know we are around. Dylan was so relaxed speaking and answering questions about himself and some hard ones of how he felt when he got breathless or couldn't do what the other kids were doing. There were a couple of times where he broke down but that was all right he wasn't used to talking about how he felt to a total stranger. It was a long afternoon but very rewarding; our boy was so strong and confident, we will always be proud of him. The doctor was excellent with him; he spoke directly with him and respected him. Dylan has a follow up with him in October.

Towards the end of August, Dylan was feeling unwell and this seemed to be happening more often, along with low saturations. We had been seeing the Paediatrician at least once a week for at least the last two months. On the night of Thursday 15 September Dylan wasn't very well. The doctor had put him on Furosemide (diuretic) as he was retaining a little fluid and his saturations were only 84% to 89%. I had called to speak to the registrar on call at the Children's Hospital and he said to increase his oxygen and to keep an eye on him and if he was no better to bring him into hospital as our paediatric cardiologist was away. The next day Dylan said, 'I think we should go and get checked out'. His year 6 camp was leaving on Monday and he desperately wanted to go. We ended up staying the Friday night and when the doctors did their rounds on Saturday morning they suggested he didn't go on the camp. 'Mum, this is my year 6 memory,' he said. 'We'll talk about it on the way home,' I said to him. We played it by ear during the weekend and on Sunday night I asked him how he was feeling and he said, 'Let's do it, even if we go for one day.' How could I say no to that! He knew his body better than I did. I rang the Principal and said, 'We're going', and she was delighted. I really didn't think it would end up being my last memory of him having so much fun.

Monday 19 September, Dylan went to Broken Bay. He was struggling the first day, finding it difficult getting to the activities so his teacher asked if they had a wheelchair. One of the guys went over to the mainland and got one; the kids took turns in pushing him around. He was able to be involved in some of the activities, but was more than happy to watch and cheer them on as well. He participated in one of the night activities where he had to get dressed up and be the daggiest kid, using the kid's clothes in his group (some very large boys in his group with very big clothes); just the rush to get changed and get to the centre where the other kids were was enough to exhaust him. After that he collapsed, he was so tired and breathless, but he did it!

On Monday 10 October Dylan had an appointment with St Vincent's so I picked him up from school after lunch. Our usual specialist wasn't there so we saw someone else. Dylan wasn't very impressed with her. 'We need to grow this boy', she said. He was very aware of his body image. She thought they should try him on a puffer equivalent to Prostacyclin, but they had to get it approved first. We were again keen to try something, as with this disease you try what you can. Unfortunately Dylan went downhill fast. That was his last day at school.

On Wednesday 12th Dylan saw his cardiologist. His feet had become very puffy and he was feeling unwell. His saturations were 86%. I borrowed a friend's wheelchair for him, which he didn't like; he was angry. I think he may have been feeling that he had no say or control over what was happening. The cardiologist sent us home and Dylan was to see the paediatrician the following week.

Dylan saw his Paediatrician on Monday 17 and Thursday 20. He was very concerned about Dylan. His tummy was so large, his feet were all puffy and he had put on seven kilograms in fluid, which Dylan thought was weight. The doctor rang the cardiologist and expressed his concerns and said that we better go to the Children's Hospital. This would have to be the first time that Dylan really argued about going to hospital. When we got home, I rang the paediatrician back and told him how adamant Dylan was about not going and he said to me, 'I'm afraid he won't last.' In all the years we had seen him he had never spoken like that. We went to the Children's Hospital, and we had a bag packed and oxygen in the car, just in case. We didn't wait too long in emergency. The nurse did Dylan's observations before he was taken to be X-rayed and have blood tests. They put him on oxygen with a mask at a 12-litre flow. His saturations were still low, but he was comfortable. The registrar spoke to me about resuscitation. Thankfully, Ayman and I had spoken about that a little while ago and we said we didn't want him resuscitated; we signed the paperwork and boy that was tough. He had gone into right heart failure.

Saturday came and he had bacon for brekky, he loved his bacon. He had a lot of visitors which was strange in itself. There were people coming to see him who had never been to visit him in hospital before and he was very tired. He managed to play Play Station with one of his friends who had been around since they were babies, Mat. Our doctor came in to talk to Dylan about going over to Manly to Bear Cottage for a visit, but Dylan wasn't wrapped in the idea (it's a place where sick kids and their families go for a little respite, a lovely place). He was comfortable but very tired, in and out of sleep. He said.'Please, Mum, not so many visitors tomorrow.' He had a disturbed sleep with a bit of coughing but the nurses looked after him so well. They gave him some extra oxygen but other than that was on no extra drugs.

Sunday morning he seemed OK. Still very tired. A couple of friends called in but didn't stay long. One of his closest friends rang to see if they could come, and Dylan was looking forward to seeing Jacob as they were like kindred spirits. Just as his mate got to the door, Dylan sat up and said he needed to be sick, he also wanted to go the toilet and he had a pain in his side. It was about 3 p.m. It all happened so fast. The nurses came in and tried to hook him up to a monitor. It was all over in about ten minutes at the most. It was the first time I had felt his heart beat slow, almost normal and I said to him as I rubbed his tummy, 'It's OK, mate, we'll be all right, you go and we'll see you later', and with that he closed his eyes.

The doctor on call passed Dylan over to Ayman. Then I held our son in my arms for the last time. He was such a brave little boy. We certainly were in shock, I didn't cry. Ayman's mum (grandma) and brother were there with us and were able to say goodbye to Dylan before he died. He was with us right to the end; for that I am thankful. Fran, Peter, Sammy and AJ came shortly after Dylan had died and they were so upset and it was like there was nothing to say. The Anglican chaplain came and she is lovely; she read the last supper, which is Dylan's favourite Bible story.

Dylan had the Lord in his heart and that was definitely evident from his peace in those last days. Dylan had such a short time with us, but he lived a full life in the time he spent with us and had many, many family and friends who loved him and miss him very much. No one will ever know what he went through, not even me. I feel privileged that we had him with us and that God chose us to look after him before he, called for him. In time the pain will start to fade but at the moment the pain in our heart is horrific.

We would like to thank all the specialists, doctors, nurses, pathologists, X-ray, home oxygen, orthopaedic team, his teachers and just everyone who was involved with us regarding Dylan and his health. You all are wonderful people and all the friends and family who have been there to help us through all the good and difficult times. I thank the Lord that we had Dylan in our lives for a short time rather than not at all. Thank you.

Leonie Ingleton

> This speech was given by Leonie Ingleton at an event to commemorate the anniversary of the first kidney transplant in Australia 40 years ago at the Queen Elizabeth Hospital. Leonie was the first 'child' to be dialysed, at 11 years of age, and the youngest person to undergo a kidney transplant. She was also the longest surviving transplant in South Australia, having had her transplant for 34 years at the time of giving this speech.

I had my kidney transplant on 20 January 1971 at the age of 13, after spending 18 months on dialysis. The transplant transformed my life.

Before my transplant I seemed to be sitting on the sidelines watching life pass me by. From about day three after the operation it was as if I stepped into the stream of life and I haven't stopped riding the current since.

Two philosophies have guided my life. The first one was that life was too short to worry about what other people thought. And the other one: how do you know you can't do something if you haven't tried?

Once I had completed my schooling I bought a car and a tent and found my freedom. I remember one of my holidays was to Wilpena Pound, where I climbed St Mary's Peak and I made sure this was recorded in my case notes at the next visit to the doctor.

In 1980 I sold my car and bought a bicycle and a piano and I resumed study. My first year at university was interrupted when I had the opportunity to participate in the 2nd International Transplant Games in New York. I came home with four silver medals for swimming. My bike was my primary mode of transport so I was very fit, but cycling was not on the list of events. I enjoyed swimming so I put my name down for that.

After the games I continued to teach swimming for six years and I still love to swim for leisure and fitness. Last year I participated in the National Transplant Games and I won a silver and three bronze medals in swimming. But my greatest triumph was winning a gold in the women's 10-kilometre bike ride.

I also used my bike for touring. When I look back on it, I find it hard to believe that I rode from Geelong to Mt Gambier along the Great Ocean Road. On another trip, I caught the train to Stawell and cycled into Halls Gap, over the Grampians and caught the train home from Horsham.

In my final year at university I met my husband, David, and within a year we were married. This didn't curb my adventures; it just meant I had someone to share them with.

Holidays have continued to bring great pleasure. Eighteen months ago my husband and I took a 14-week trip around Australia. I love the outdoors and more recently have found it to be the inspiration for my paintings. I have been painting for eleven years now and find it is my way of giving expression to my experiences and gratitude for life.

My transplanted kidney had a 50% chance of surviving the first year. I have never taken life for granted and I have felt that each day is a bonus. Years ago I used to ponder if I would see the new millennium in and I have. What has the transplant meant to me? The chance to have a life, and a very good one at that. I am 47 years of age and I have had my transplant for 34 of them.

My story would have been a very different story if it weren't for the family who gave consent to organ donation at a very difficult time when a family member had died. That's a decision they made many years ago and that kidney is still doing its thing silently and sweetly. The miracle really does begin with the donor family.

Before I close, I want to thank those who have given their support and expert medical care through TQEH over all these years. Without this I would not have been able to accomplish what I have. My hope is that I am a living testament to what medical science can achieve, offer hope to those awaiting a transplant and give encouragement to recipients to make the most of their 'gift of life'.

Ebony Keys (poem to an organ donor)
- Mel Rees

At times my hope seems to fade,
like the sun in the evening sky,
but you remind me life is not so dark,
and make night-time a lighter shade.
for although we will never meet,
I am living my life for two.
In times of darkness,
you are my morning light.
At times life's songs seem so sombre,
and all I play are ebony keys,
but you remind me of happier tunes,
and the melody seems much stronger.
For although we will never meet,
I am living my life for two.
When my songs are dark,
you are my keys of white.

www.ingramcontent.com/pod-product-compliance
Lightning Source LLC
Chambersburg PA
CBHW071117030426
42336CB00013BA/2132